Natural
Mothering

Natural Mothering

A Guide to Holistic Therapies for Pregnancy,
Birth, and Early Childhood

NICKY WESSON

ILLUSTRATIONS BY VATSALA SPERLING
PHOTOGRAPHS BY SUZANNE ARMS

Healing Arts Press
Rochester, Vermont

Healing Arts Press
One Park Street
Rochester, Vermont 05767
www.gotoit.com

*Note to the reader: This book is intended as an informational guide. The remedies,
approaches, and techniques described herein are meant to supplement, and not to be a
substitute for, professional medical care or treatment. They should not be used to treat a
serious ailment without prior consultation with a qualified health-care professional.*

Library of Congress Cataloging-in-Publication Data
Wesson, Nicky.
    [Alternative maternity]
    Natural mothering : a guide to holistic therapies for pregnancy, birth, and
early childhood / Nicky Wesson.
        p.   cm.
    Previously published in London by Macdonald Optima in 1989 under
the title: Alternative maternity.
    Includes bibliographical references and index.
    ISBN 0-89281-733-X (alk. paper)
    1. Pregnancy. 2. Childbirth. 3. Infants (Newborn)—Care. 4. Alternative
medicine. I. Title.
RG525.W566   1997   97-10399
618.2'4—dc21   CIP

Printed and bound in Canada

10 9 8 7 6 5 4 3 2 1

Special thanks to Sandra and Molly Dickin for excellent and agreeable modeling

Type design and layout by Peri Champine
This book was typeset in Columbus

Healing Arts Press is a division of Inner Traditions International

Contents

Part 3—Caring for Your Baby

Acknowledgments

I thank all of the following who have given generously of their time to help me write this book: Jane Arnold, Gwen Attwood, Caroline and Eleanor Casteron, Paul and Sally Dean, Sara Drake, Marie Fauré-Anderson, Sue Francia, Christine Grabowska, Harriet Griffey, Heather Guerini, Christine Hall, Anne Mamok, Jane May, Christine Meadows, Dorothy Norris, Rosamund Parker, Vicki Pitman, Keki Sidwa, Adrian Stoddart, Pat Taylor, David Raitt, Val Thomas, Heather Welford, and Angela Yates. I would particularly like to thank Linda Razzell to whom I am indebted for the information on homeopathy.

Preface to the Third Edition

Alternative remedies and therapies are becoming more widely accepted, offering a greater range of solutions for the physical problems that beset people. Fortunately, there are signs that doctors are starting to be aware of the advantages of complementary medicine and referring their patients or taking the training themselves. Doubtless contributing to its acceptance are patient demand and the fact that such treatment may not only be more successful and safer than drug therapy, but it can be much cheaper. Research is needed now more than ever so that we can regain the knowledge that has been lost and benefit from it, while gaining a more accurate idea of its efficacy and limitations.

Change in the area of childbirth is evident from the way in which midwives and visiting nurses in Britain now recommend homeopathic Arnica to be taken prophylactically around the time of birth. Although there are doubtless still some skeptics, women no longer feel that they have to take such remedies surreptitiously and are freer to care for themselves.

Having access to information about alternative approaches enables women to exert some control over what happens to them rather than passively putting their well-being in the hands of medical and midwifery staff. One example of the way in which women can improve their chances of giving birth with the minimum of difficulty is promoted by Jean Sutton whose work is just becoming established in Britain. Jean is a New Zealand midwife with many years of experience. She has observed that it is possible for women to influence the position of their babies before labor starts so that when it does, the baby is in the best possible position (left occiput anterior) in which to pass through the pelvis. Her theory is that postures adopted by pregnant women as the consequence of modern living predispose babies to adopt unfavorable positions in the uterus. This results in a higher incidence of forceps, vacuum extraction, and cesarean section deliveries, and a greater number of inductions of labor with increased need for pain relief.

Optimal fetal positioning should be adopted from thirty-two weeks of pregnancy for the first baby and for the last two to three weeks in women who have already had children. It involves being careful never to sit so that your knees are higher than your hips nor to slouch backward—positions that are hard to avoid in modern sofas or car seats. It is best either to sit completely upright with a straight back and knees level with hips or adopt any position such as leaning or kneeling forward over cushions or a bean bag, sitting on an orthopedic stool, or any other position that tips the pelvis forward so that the area available for the baby's head to enter the pelvis is increased. The best position in which to sleep is lying propped on your left side or, if possible, on or leaning toward your front.

I was particularly interested in the possibility of optimal fetal positioning because all of my children except one have been malpositioned— from being merely posterior to a face presentation, including one who presented ear first. As a result, I was glad to be able to do something that might mean my last baby's birth would be more straightforward. Although his head did not engage before labor started, he was in the right position when it did and was born at home without difficulty.

A further happy example of influencing birth events comes from Jan Hibbert whose previous labor is described in my book *Home Birth*. Her last baby was born four days overdue, following a long, hard labor. He weighed twelve pounds and had problems being delivered because his shoulders became stuck in the pelvis. Fearing a repetition with the next baby, Jan used acupuncture and homeopathic and herbal remedies to start labor early and make it easier. This morning, a few days before her baby was due, she gave birth to an eleven-pound baby girl, Lydia. She had a three-hour labor and needed no stitches, proving that it is possible to swing things your way.

Preface to the Second Edition

In the five years since I wrote this book the climate regarding alternative medicine has changed considerably. Use of alternative remedies has become far more common, with the use of aromatherapy and homeopathy almost becoming commonplace. The change in attitude has brought with it a greater recognition that mothers have both the right and the responsibility to choose how they and their children are treated. Mothers are growing more confident about trusting their instincts and listening to the voice that tells them they do know best about themselves and their babies.

My children continue to do well on home remedies—the younger three (there is another!) have still managed to overcome illnesses without ever using antibiotics.

In the last two years, many more of the mothers I meet are actively interested in hearing about alternatives. Some have tried these therapies, often as a last resort, and have become convinced that these treatments have worked for them when everything else has failed. It is particularly rewarding to be able to recommend medical herbalism for treatment of recurrent miscarriages for example, or reflexology for infertility, and see women with babies that they would otherwise have been unlikely to have had.

From major successes such as solving infertility or miscarriage to the minor but no less significant help with problems of morning sickness or sleeplessness in babies, offering a solution that works is enormously satisfying and is why I feel I can recommend even more positively the benefits of trying alternatives.

Preface to the First Edition

When my first child was born eleven years ago, I was completely wedded to the medical model. It had simply never occurred to me to do anything other than go to a doctor when ill. My daughter Alicia was born in a hospital and returned there five weeks later with a problem that remained undiagnosed. She had severe colic, was frequently ill, and consumed pints of antibiotics. She had a couple of operations as a result of constant ear infections and, understandably, was not always a happy child. My next child, Duncan, was born after a complicated labor and an emergency cesarean section. He too had constant ear infections, eczema, and, we eventually discovered, an allergy to milk, wheat, and eggs. Hospital care, a very restricted diet, and drugs kept both Alicia and Duncan reasonably well, but not without difficulties, side effects, and a feeling of unease at having such young children on constant medication.

In 1984 when our third child, Alastair, was a few months old, I attended a conference that was to revolutionize our lives. The topic was alternative medicine for pregnancy, labor, and babies, and it covered acupuncture, homeopathy, herbalism, and osteopathy. I knew at once that this holistic approach might offer solutions to the problems we were still struggling with. Alastair was proving more severely allergic;

we even had to drop out of a double-blind trial testing breastfed babies who had eczema because he reacted so badly to allergens in my breast milk whenever I had eggs or milk.

Not without misgivings, I took him to acupuncturist Adrian Stoddart, who had given the lecture. He applied acupressure to him, and literally overnight his food sensitivity decreased. Due partly to luck and partly to my newly gained knowledge that I enthusiastically put into practice, both Alastair and his younger sister, Octavia, have never taken an anti-biotic. Cranial osteopathy on the two older children who both had instrumental deliveries has put a stop to their ear infections and has made them far happier. It has even obviated the need for my eleven-year-old to have four of her adult teeth removed and wear braces. Octavia, now two, was treated for colic soon after birth and has since remained sunny and relaxed. Having osteopathic treatment myself before the birth meant that she almost shot out, in sharp contrast to my difficult previous labors.

Acupuncture has improved the health of myself and my children enormously; we use herbs to treat infection and have used homeopathy and hypnotherapy on occasion with success. Through recommending these alternatives to others, I know that we are not alone in finding that they provide answers to problems that do not respond to conventional remedies.

Of course, such alternatives are not infallible, the treatment is not free, and we are still grateful for traditional medical and hospital care when necessary. However, it is wonderful that such occasions are now so few and far between. As a result of my experiences, I have compiled the information to provide you with the knowledge that I wish I'd had as a new parent.

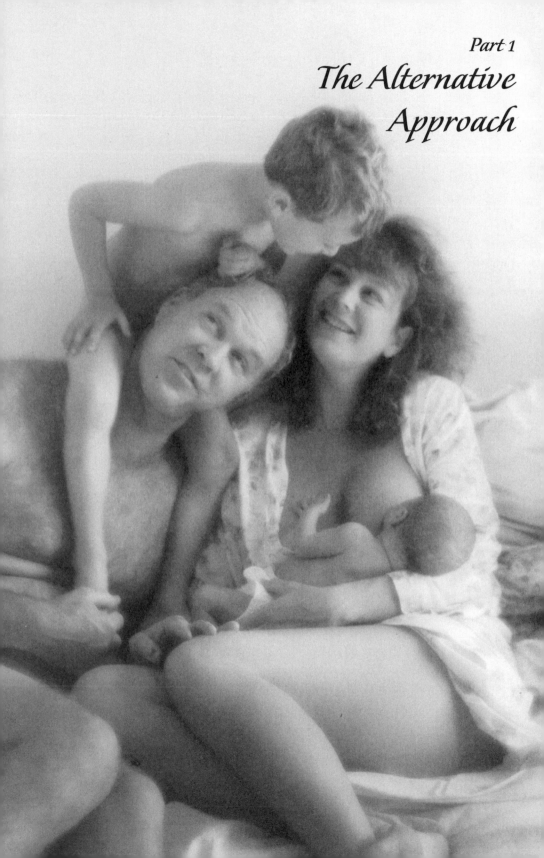

1

Why Try an Alternative Therapy?

The first questions to be answered in a book like this are, Why should I use alternatives, what can they do for me that my doctor cannot, and are they safe for pregnant mothers and their babies?

The prime reason for choosing to use an alternative approach to any specific health problem is its superior scope. There are many examples of people being cured of ailments for which either there is no equivalent treatment in orthodox medicine or there is a treatment but it has either not proved effective or is likely to be risky or have side effects. For instance, homeopathic treatment before birth can prevent the baby from inheriting health problems. Acupuncture can cure infertility when orthodox treatment has failed. Cranial osteopathy can remedy pyloric stenosis, a potentially dangerous condition in which babies repeatedly vomit their entire feed, by working through the outside of the baby's head as opposed to abdominal operation, which is the conventional answer.

Practitioners of alternative medicine aim to enable the body to heal itself. The treatment is of you as a whole and will take into consideration your diet, lifestyle, and feelings about your problem. Although you are only likely to seek help if you have a particular need, their aim is to assist your body to function at its best, so that a preconception visit can be a sensible step.

Alternative remedies are particularly suited to those who actively want to accept responsibility for the health of themselves and their children. A growing number of people prefer to treat themselves with natural remedies, learning which remedies suit them, and saving antibiotics for life-threatening emergencies. Such people may find the active medical management of modern obstetrics particularly inappropriate and damaging and prefer to assume control of the situation themselves. For them and the midwives who share their belief in the body's ability to give birth without medical intervention, I have included some of the remedies to ease childbirth that have been used for many years.

Such remedies are not harmless in the sense of being ineffectual, but they are safe to take in the way described. Since the thalidomide disaster, women have rightly been very cautious about taking any drug during pregnancy, and indeed it is usually best to allow your body the opportunity to heal itself. However there are situations, such as with morning sickness, in which a remedy is desired. This book offers a range of remedies, with a wider selection for the more common problems. This should make it possible for you to choose a remedy that works for you and, whenever possible, is readily available and inexpensive. However, it is important to point out that it is wise to seek help from a practitioner for long-standing or serious problems.

Perhaps the best way to find a good alternative therapist is by word of mouth because many therapies can treat a variety of problems, and it may be better to choose the person rather than the therapy. However, some types of problems are best suited to particular modalities, for instance back and spine problems to osteopathy or chiropractic. There may also be other factors to bear in mind when making your choice. Some people, for example, are apprehensive about needles and so dislike the idea of acupuncture, while others may be limited by what is available in their area.

If you have not heard of anyone suitable, write to the respective professional body for a list of their members. Then call the nearest practitioner, outline your problem, and see if you can get a rough idea of how many treatments you might require. Price can be a drawback, so don't be hesitant about asking about the fees. These can vary widely, although many therapists say that they would prefer to reduce their fees rather than send someone in urgent need of treatment away. There is often a reduction for children, whom many therapists particularly enjoy treating, because they respond so well and rapidly to treatment. Find out whether they are prepared to prescribe over the phone once they know you. A good practitioner should know his or her limitations and be able to refer you to someone else if they are not able to help.

It can be very refreshing to have an unhurried consultation with a therapist, and you should feel that the improvement in your health makes it worth every penny.

2

A Guide to
Alternative
Therapies

ACUPUNCTURE

This is a complete system of medicine that was developed in China
five thousand years ago. It is based on the theory that the body
consists of two opposing energetic forces, yin and yang. Yin is deep,
cold, and feminine, and yang is hot, stimulating, male, and related
to the sun. In good health yin and yang are perfectly balanced, but in illness this balance is disturbed.

An acupuncturist will make a diagnosis by taking a full
history from you and also by noting your appearance, color,
and smell. He or she will then feel your pulses. An acupuncturist can detect as many as fourteen separate pulses,
and each one reveals potential imbalances within your body.
Traditional Chinese medicine proposes that the organs of the
body are connected by invisible pathways of energy, so that illness in a particular organ may cause pain to be felt in another
place along its particular energy pathway or meridian. It is held
that illness is caused by obstruction of the energy that should be

flowing along these channels and that insertion of the acupuncture needles removes the blockage and allows energy to flow freely again.

The treatment consists of having several very fine needles inserted into different parts of your body for a period of about half an hour. The needles only hurt briefly as they are inserted. Sometimes the acupuncturist may rotate the needles, or send a weak electric current through them. Sometimes dried mugwort or moxa is burned so that heat is transmitted through the needle or directly warms the skin. Once the treatment has been completed, your pulses are checked to ensure that the treatment has been effective. You may feel light-headed or sleepy afterward. Depending on your need, you may be offered dietary advice and be given further treatments.

The benefits of acupuncture are that no drugs are used and that its scope is far broader than that of Western medicine. Some of its applications are especially suited to pregnancy, for example turning breech babies or inducing labor without drugs. Acupuncture is also a superior system of treatment because it frequently proves effective where no orthodox treatment has succeeded, as in some cases of infertility or recurrent miscarriage.

AROMATHERAPY

This is the use of essential plant oils to stimulate, soothe, refresh, and heal. The oils are pure distillations from plants and are very concentrated. Some of them have antiseptic properties.

They can be used in various ways, but all of them involve some form of dilution, because they can harm the skin if applied neat. You can add a few drops to your bath, put drops onto a handkerchief, add a little to a bowl of warm water to scent a room, or take a minute amount on a cube of sugar. The oils are often used in massage, when they are diluted in a ratio of one drop of essential oil to one-half teaspoonful (2 ml) of a vegetable oil such as olive or almond. They can also be added to hot water and used as a compress. They are especially suitable for pregnancy and labor.

You can buy the oils from most health food stores or order them by mail. Oils that should be avoided in pregnancy (because they may cause miscarriage) are basil, clove, hyssop, marjoram, and myrrh. Oils that should never be used at home include origanum, sage, savory, thyme, and wintergreen.

For baths make up a 6 percent blend, i.e., six drops of essential oil per teaspoon (5 ml) of base, which can be whole milk or vodka (for babies and very young children, use two to three drops of essential oil per teaspoon of carrier). The oil needs to be dispersed with a carrier or you may get neat oil on your skin, which can sting or irritate it. If your bath is made of fiberglass or plastic, it is important to wipe the oil off after the bath.

Oils that should be avoided in pregnancy are:
ajowan, aniseed, basil, birch, bitter almond, baldo, buchu, camphor, clove, cornmint, fennel (all types), horseradish, hyssop, lavender, cotton, *Lavendula stoechas*, mugwort, mustard, myrrh, oregano, parsley seed, pennyroyal, *Pimenta racemosa*, plecanthrus, rue, *Salvia officianalis*, sassafras, savin, savory, star aniseed, tansy, tarragon, thuja, thyme (thymol type), wintergreen, wormseed, wormwood.

People who suffer from epilepsy should not use fennel, sage, or hyssop essential oils. People who have high blood pressure should avoid using fennel, hyssop, sage, and thyme oils.

BACH FLOWER REMEDIES

In 1930 Dr. Edward Bach discovered thirty-eight different flower remedies. Each one is derived from a flower that has been floated on water in a glass bowl in full sun. The water is preserved with an equal amount of brandy and bottled. Dr. Bach discovered that these remedies had very beneficial effects on negative states of the mind, such as timidity, guilt, lack of confidence, fearfulness, or exhaustion.

The remedies are now available from most health food stores, and you can treat yourself with the aid of Dr. Bach's booklet, *The Twelve*

Healers, or one of the other available guides. You may use more than one remedy at the same time, either putting two drops of each into a glass of water or fruit juice or by making up a solution with two tablespoons (30 ml) of water and taking four drops on the tongue. Add a teaspoonful (5 ml) of brandy or cider vinegar if you want the mixture to keep for more than three weeks. The remedies should be taken at least four times per day.

Rescue Remedy is a combination of five flower remedies—Star of Bethlehem, Rock Rose, Impatiens, Cherry Plum, and Clematis. It is extremely useful in cases of mental and physical shock, terror, panic, or trauma. Take four drops in water if possible or apply to the lips and the pulse points on the wrists and behind the ears.

Cranial Osteopathy

Cranial osteopaths are qualified osteopaths who specialize in working on your whole body via the fluid and membranes of your brain and spinal cord. They find that by working on the skull, they can assess the state of the connective tissue throughout your body and see where old traumas are preventing it from functioning properly. They are then able to remove the impediments that prevent those areas moving in time with the body's internal fluid tide. Correcting them will enable you to function with a good flow of energy and feeling of well-being and ensure that your body's involuntary mechanisms are working well. Such treatment is especially valuable for pregnant women and babies.

The treatment consists of lying on a couch for forty minutes while your head is held firmly. You may feel pressure and perhaps subtle changes within it, but it is not painful. You may feel slightly giddy for a few seconds afterward.

Pregnancy is an especially good time to be treated cranially because the altered hormone levels and changes in the endocrine system make the connective tissues much softer and more fluid and so better able to alter. The treatment will release any compression in the pelvis, enabling it to stretch fully during the birth. The osteopath will also be working on the sacral nerves that influence the pelvis, cervix, and perineum, balancing them so that the cervix dilates smoothly. He or she may also work directly on the pelvis. This treatment is particularly beneficial to women who have had difficulty in giving birth.

Cranial treatment can be extremely useful in treating babies too. The pressures that are exerted on their heads during birth are very great and can cause the membranes to shear and become twisted. This may be obvious if the head is very molded or looks asymmetrical. Obviously, difficult births are potentially damaging, but even quick and easy births can stress the cranial mechanism. There is a case for suggesting that all babies should receive treatment fourteen days after the birth, even those born by elective cesarean section, because they will have missed the benefits of the rhythmic squeezing and elastic recoil of birth that stimulates pulmonary respiration and gets the temporal bones moving.

In some cultures grandmothers routinely massage the babies' heads to make them nicely rounded and well-shaped; people from these cultures have a lower than average incidence of psychological and personality problems.

You may want to take your baby for treatment if he or she is crying a lot, failing to sleep, hyperactive, or frequently sick. Babies do try to help themselves by attempting to expand their palates and open up their cranial mechanisms by means of crying, thumb-sucking, and yawning, but they need help. Cranial work can make a miraculous difference to them, often overnight, even to children well past babyhood. It can be especially beneficial for children who are mentally handicapped.

Abigail was born with Down syndrome and two holes in the heart. She was treated by a cranial osteopath twice a week for four months from birth and then seen weekly for another couple of months. The holes in her heart closed spontaneously, and she is said to be at the top of the intelligence range for a Down's child. Her features still show signs of the syndrome but are not at all marked. Her medical attendants are amazed at how well she has done.

HERBAL MEDICINE

Herbs have been used for thousands of years as a gentle and effective way of relieving symptoms and improving general health. They harmonize the body's metabolic processes and correct imbalances within them. Each whole plant is balanced so that often there are elements within it that protect the user from any potentially harmful side effects of the active constituents. Taking the whole plant or plant part is a far safer method of using its healing properties than that employed by modern pharmaceuticals, in which drugs are frequently obtained from herbs, but the constituents are isolated and so are without the protective qualities of the rest of the plant.

Herbs do have a physiological effect and so it is best whenever possible to consult a medical herbalist, who will have had extensive training about the appropriate remedy for your particular needs. He or she will take a detailed history and may give you dietary advice. However, herbs have been used safely by ordinary people for many centuries, and you may want to try some gentle ones yourself. Some herbs should be avoided in pregnancy; these include aloe vera, autumn crocus, barberry, broom, juniper, pennyroyal, pokeroot, parsley, southernwood, tansy, thuja, wormwood, feverfew, and sassafras. Goldenseal should not be taken during pregnancy, although it is very useful for stimulating contractions once labor begins.

There are a number of ways of preparing herbs. You can use them fresh or dried or buy them in a concentrated fluid form such as extracts or tinctures. They can also be obtained as powders, which are used to make poultices and pastes or put into capsules for swallowing. Herbs are also made into ointments.

If you are preparing herbs at home, it is easiest to make either a decoction or an infusion. An infusion or tea is made from the aerial parts of a plant—the leaves, stalks, or flowers. It is prepared by putting one teaspoonful of the dried herb or three teaspoonfuls of the fresh herb into a container, and pouring on a cupful of boiling water. This should then be covered and allowed to stand for fifteen minutes without further heating. Strain and drink it while still warm. A decoction is made from the hard parts of plants, such as the roots, rhizomes, or stems, which need to be boiled to release their medicinal qualities. Cut or crush the herb as much as possible before putting it into a stainless steel or enamel saucepan. Add cold water—one pint (600 ml) to one ounce (25 g) of dried herb, three ounces (75 g) of fresh—bring it to a boil and simmer it for fifteen minutes or more. Remove it from the heat and allow it to infuse; then strain and drink it warm.

Infusions and decoctions should be used within twenty-four hours. They can be gently reheated to a temperature below boiling and may be sweetened with honey or made more palatable by the addition of licorice root.

Extracts and tinctures are herbal preparations that have been distilled with water and alcohol respectively. They are very concentrated, so dose may vary from a drop or two (in the case of very potent herbs) to five to fifteen drops.

HOMEOPATHY

This is a method of enabling the body to heal itself discovered by Samuel Hahnemann, a German, in 1796. He found that giving minute doses of the drugs that caused symptoms identical to those of the disease being treated actually cured the condition. This established the principle of homeopathy which is "let like be cured by like." The symptoms of illness are seen as the reaction of the body in its attempts to overcome the disease. Homeopathic remedies help the body by strengthening the reaction and allowing the body to heal itself.

For accurate diagnosis and treatment, you need to visit a homeopath, who will take a detailed history of your illness and want to know a lot of details about you, what makes you feel better or worse, what kind of temperament you have, your likes and dislikes, and so forth, before prescribing a remedy. The remedy chosen will be specifically for you, so that you will receive a different remedy than someone else with the same complaint. You can only be sure of getting the correct remedy by visiting a homeopath, although you may be able to consult by phone after the initial visit. For serious or long-standing complaints, a proper consultation is essential. However, a number of the more common remedies are now widely available, and you may want to try them for yourself. If the remedy fails, it is often because the wrong one has been chosen.

The remedies are available in different strengths; unlike orthodox drugs, the strongest are the most dilute. There are thousands of remedies, prepared largely from plants, although some are made from substances that are regarded as inert, such as gold and sand. They are prepared by serial dilution from a mother tincture. This means that one drop of the tincture is diluted with nine or ninety-nine drops of the diluting medium, depending on whether the potency is to be decimal (x) or centesimal (c). The mixture is shaken vigorously, and then one drop from that mixture is taken and diluted again in the same ratio. The first dilution becomes 1x or c, the second 2x or c, etc. The potency generally available is 6x, which is the potency most suitable for self-administration. The x is often omitted so that a remedy might appear as Hepar sulph. 6, for example.

A combination remedy composed of Aconite, Belladonna, and Chamomilla, ABC tablets should be part of every family's homeopathic first aid kit; ABC tablets can be administered after bumps and falls and at the start of any childhood illness.

Using the Remedies

To use a remedy take one tablet three times a day for two to three days. In acute conditions take a tablet six times a day, and for very painful conditions such as earache you may need to dose yourself every fifteen minutes. When you start to improve, increase the interval between the doses until the improvement is established and then stop. Sometimes the remedy will seem to make the condition worse, in which case stop it altogether. This will probably be followed by a significant improvement. Only restart the remedy if the symptoms recur.

In urgent or high energy conditions, such as a fever or labor, remedies can be given every five, ten, or fifteen minutes as needed. You should generally only take one remedy at a time, and avoid other medicines because they may detract from the remedy's efficiency.

The remedies come as tablets or powders, which should be allowed to dissolve under the tongue. They should be taken in a clean mouth, which means you should not have anything to eat or drink for a half hour before or after taking the remedy. Avoid coffee and peppermint while you are using homeopathy, because they may act as antidotes. This may mean you will need to buy one of the toothpastes designed for homeopathy users. You should also avoid using essential oils of black pepper, camphor, eucalyptus, or the mints as they can antidote the effects of homeopathy.

The medicines are sensitive and can easily become contaminated, so you must store them in a cool, dark place away from strong smells. Keep them in their original containers, and tip the pills out into the lid so that you do not touch any that you need to put back. If you drop any, do not put the spilled ones back into the bottle. The remedies can also be taken in warm water; this is particularly suitable for acute conditions where doses need to be taken frequently. Crush two tablets and dissolve in warm water.

Babies can be given tablets powdered, either dry or in a little water, or you can put a tablet inside the cheek of a sleeping child.

REFLEXOLOGY

This is another method of bringing about changes in the body by applying pressure on an apparently unrelated area. It dates back to 3000 B.C. in China and has been practiced widely in countries as far apart as Egypt and Japan for thousands of years.

Reflexologists believe that all parts of the body have corresponding areas on the feet and hands, and they find they are able to treat a problem in the body by applying pressure to the relevant area on the feet. It is particularly suited for problems such as back pain, allergies, insomnia, sinusitis, constipation, asthma, and stress-induced illness. It has had some notable success in treating infertility.

Treatment lasts about an hour and starts with a gentle exploratory massage of all areas of both feet. The practitioner may ask for details of your history first or prefer to discover the problem by examining you. Reflexologists feel for gritty lumps under the skin in the areas that represent the areas of disease, and they then apply pressure to these points in a way that may be tender or even painful. The treatment may leave you feeling tired, but you should notice an improvement immediately or within several sessions.

Reflexology is not recommended during the first trimester of pregnancy or if you have bleeding or a history of miscarriage.

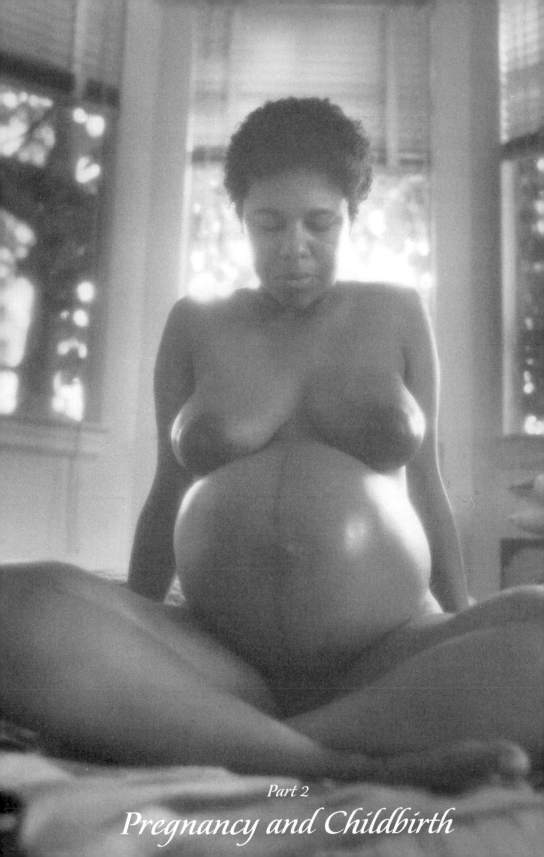

Part 2
Pregnancy and Childbirth

3

Planning for Pregnancy

Many people conceive unintentionally and many others cannot conceive when they want to, so there are a lot of people for whom the question of timing or preparing for pregnancy is irrelevant. However, there are ways in which you can make sure that the baby you are planning to have is as healthy as possible, some of which may not be obvious or may require a change of lifestyle. It is well worth considering because taking care of yourself before and during pregnancy does actually make a difference to the health and strength of your baby and can make the difference between a miserable pregnancy and an enjoyable one.

Provided conception does not prove a problem, you may want to consider the following:

- When would you want the baby to be born? Winter babies can be fun if you feel that you are going to be quite happy staying in when the baby is very small, but the amount of wrapping and unwrapping involved can also be a deterrent to getting out and may mean that you end up feeling isolated. Summer babies need less wrapping but may mean that you are pregnant in the heat, which can be enervating.

- Will you lose maternity benefits or your entitlement to maternity leave if you become pregnant now rather than in a few months time? Insurance and employment rules change, and you should find out how they apply to you before you become pregnant.
- If you already have children in school or day care, will you be in the early months of the pregnancy, when you are likely to feel most tired, during the holidays? Will the baby be due during the holidays and is this an advantage or not?
- March conceptions can be Christmas babies. It is worth thinking about the baby's birthday and subsequent parties, which are usually much easier if there is a chance that they can be held outside.
- If you plan to move or renovate the house while pregnant—a surprising number of people do—can you avoid it happening in the early or late months of the pregnancy?

PRECONCEPTUAL CARE

A list of health considerations for a planned pregnancy includes:

- Stop taking the contraceptive pill at least three months before trying to get pregnant. Some as yet unsubstantiated studies suggest there is a higher risk of defects, such as cleft palate, in babies conceived immediately after stopping the pill.
- Pay attention to your daily food intake, avoiding refined foods such as cookies, cakes, sweets, high-fat foods like chips, and foods that contain large amounts of sugar, additives, and artificial colorings. Eat fresh rather than prepared foods, concentrating on meat, fish, cheese, whole grains, pulses, fruits, and vegetables. If you are a vegetarian make sure that you are tak-

ing a vitamin B_{12} supplement and maybe a multivitamin. Also avoid eating raw or undercooked meats, and do not drink unpasteurized milk or eat soft cheeses.

- Avoid, or at least reduce, the use of alcohol and cigarettes. Smoking affects the baby directly, giving rise to babies of lower birth weight who may be born prematurely, suffer the consequences of pregnancy complications, and be susceptible to respiratory infections after birth. It can also increase the miscarriage rate and is responsible for poor physical and mental growth in babies born to smokers.[1] Smoking has been shown to halve the success rate of in vitro fertilization, which suggests that if you are having problems conceiving, you should stop or reduce smoking.[2]

- Alcohol should be avoided, especially around the time of conception and during pregnancy, particularly in the first three months. Alcohol addiction in a pregnant woman can lead to fetal alcohol syndrome in which the baby has distinctive facial features and is likely to be mentally retarded. The safe limit for alcohol is not known and is likely to vary between individuals, so it is simplest to avoid it altogether if possible or for at least the first three months of pregnancy. Acupuncture can help treat addictions.

- Get fit—by swimming, cycling, or some other type of all-round exercise. Pregnancy makes considerable demands on the body and labor itself can take a significant physical toll. Both can be easier if you start off in good shape.

- Try to get any long-standing problems cleared up; these might include systemic candida (see page 88), allergies, and so on. If you think there may be any type of inherited defect that could be passed on to your children, it would be wise to seek some genetic counseling. Some of these types of problems can be treated homeopathically.

- Stop any drugs that are not essential. You may need to discuss this with your doctor or midwife or seek advice from a prenatal clinic. It may also be worth consulting an alternative practitioner if you have a problem for which you need to take drugs during pregnancy. There is always the chance that you can be treated effectively so that you no longer require the drugs. Avoid drugs such as aspirin too.

- Try to cut out tea and coffee and other caffeine-containing substances, such a chocolate and cola, which may be harmful to the fetus. Recent research shows that women who are finding it difficult to conceive should cut down on coffee.[3] More than three cups of coffee a day doubles the chances of conception being delayed by a year.

- Be careful not to get overheated. There is some evidence that taking long hot baths or using an electric blanket in the early months of pregnancy can increase the risk of miscarriage, as can smoking and drinking alcohol.

- It has been known for some time that taking folic acid supplements in the three months before conception and in the first thirty days of pregnancy can reduce the likelihood of having a baby who suffers from spina bifida or anencephaly. Food rich in folic acid include vegetables (especially brussels sprouts, potatoes, spinach); fruits such as oranges and orange juice; and all cereals. If you wish to take a supplement, the recommended dosage is 0.4 mg.

- Check your rubella status by having a blood test done to see whether you are immune to German measles. If you are not, then have the immunization, but be sure to allow three months between having the immunization and trying to conceive.

- Avoid environmental hazards as much as possible; these include insecticides and herbicides. Also, watch out for lead fumes from stripping old paint; hair spray and dyes; mercury amalgam at the dentist; cooking with aluminum; medication if it can be avoided, including treatment for threadworms and lice; and radiation from X rays and, debatably, video display units. A general proviso would be to avoid anything that makes you feel ill or that you intuitively feel will not be good for your baby.

- Pregnant women should avoid contact with sheep that are lambing because of the risk of acquiring an infection that can cause miscarriage in humans.

Obviously, you will sometimes be unable to avoid some of these hazards, and clearly instinct does not work for everyone, particularly for those whose addictions overwhelm their intuition. However, most women find that even in very early pregnancy they avoid things that are potentially damaging. Alcohol, cigarettes, and coffee frequently cause nausea, and one should obey these instincts. Women sometimes find other foods that are less obviously harmful intolerable too, such as fatty and spicy foods. It can be equally surprising to find yourself craving foods that you normally dislike. Providing they are not obviously damaging, you can indulge these instincts.

The first thirteen to fourteen weeks of pregnancy are those in which the baby's organs and limbs are being formed, and these are the weeks in which it is most important to avoid exposure to anything that could cause the baby to be malformed. The time around conception is thought to be especially important. Since it is not until your period is due that you can confirm a pregnancy, this means being careful from *before* ovulation onward.

4

Problems with Conceiving

As many as one in six couples has problems with fertility, although a problem is usually recognized as existing only when conception has not occurred after at least a year of trying. The causes range from the mechanical, such as scar tissue as a consequence of pelvic disease or a complete absence of sperm, to unexplained infertility in which tests show that everything is functioning well and yet pregnancy does not occur.

Some problems can only be treated by surgery. For instance, if both fallopian tubes are blocked, it is unlikely that alternative treatments will help. However, alternative treatments *do* treat infertility successfully in many cases where orthodox treatment has failed.

Any couple failing to become pregnant should first look at their diet and lifestyle and see if there is room for improvement. Although it is quite possible to become pregnant on a very limited diet and while under great stress, these conditions can cause infertility in some individuals. Lifestyle is also an area that tends to be ignored by infertility clinics, so that you could be attending the clinic for months while living on coffee and lettuce leaves, your stress level pushed ever higher by all the tension and anguish commonly felt by those seeking treatment. An inadequate diet, and even a good one, may not be providing some of the trace elements that can be essential for conception. Even those eating well may, for some reason of individual metabolism, be deficient in some elements.

Supplements suggested by Dr. Stephen Davies and Dr. Alan Stewart in their comprehensive book, *Nutritional Medicine* (Pan, 1987), are as follows.

For Women

Follow dietary advice in Chapter 3. Take a broad spectrum multivitamin and mineral supplement and vitamin E (200 to 400 I.U. daily, though Susun Weed suggests that 500 to 1,500 I.U. taken daily can prevent birth defects in children of couples who have had previous children with birth defects).

For Men

Daily doses of:

> Multivitamin and mineral supplement
> Elemental zinc (50 mg)
> Vitamin C (200 to 500 mg)
> Lysine (500 mg)
> Arginine (1.5 to 2 g)
> Free-form amino acids (500 mg twice daily)
> Vitamin E (200 to 400 I.U., see above).

Conventional treatment starts by checking that ovulation is taking place, so if you are considering seeing your doctor because of fertility problems, it is a good idea to chart your basal body temperature (see page 33 for details of how to go about doing this). If ovulation is not occurring even though you may be having periods, it can be induced with various alternative therapies or, as a last resort, with drugs. Excessive exercise can prevent ovulation.

A sperm count can be run fairly readily, and this will show whether there are adequate numbers of sperm and whether they are healthy and able to move freely. A low sperm count is less easily treated, although lowering the temperature of the testicles by bathing them in cool water, wearing boxer shorts, and losing weight if overweight can help because the testes need to be cool to function properly.

If ovulation is taking place and the sperm count is adequate, the next step is likely to be laparoscopy, the internal examination of the woman's pelvic cavity by means of a fiber-optic telescope inserted through a small incision made just below the navel. This is done under general anesthetic. With the help of the laparoscope, the surgeon can see if there are adhesions caused by pelvic infection or endometriosis, a condition caused by tissue from the lining of the uterus growing outside it, yet bleeding monthly and forming cysts. Adhesions can mean the fallopian tubes are not free to move to scoop up the egg, that their ends are stuck together, or that they are affected in some way that prevents fertilization from taking place. Tubes can be tested for blockage by filling the uterus with dye and examining its progress up the tubes on an X ray. An alternative test is to blow air through the tubes.

One or more of these tests may reveal a problem that can only be corrected with surgery or complex techniques such as in vitro fertilization. However, most infertile couples have no evident impediment to conception, and for them the following alternative treatments may result in pregnancy.

ALTERNATIVE TREATMENTS FOR INFERTILITY

Acupuncture

There have been some remarkable successes with acupuncture to treat both male and female infertility. An acupuncturist treats you individually and may advise you about diet. Acupuncture can also help women who conceive easily but miscarry repeatedly.

Lindsay sought the help of an acupuncturist because she had glandular fever and low blood pressure, which resulted in frequent fainting. She had been trying to get pregnant for eighteen months but with no success. The blood pressure problem was alleviated by the first treatment, and subsequently her periods were regularized and her ovarian cysts dispersed. She had acupuncture monthly at ovulation to strengthen her body's reactions and to make her fit to maintain a pregnancy. Her husband had acupuncture to improve a low sperm count, and within two months she was pregnant. She had treatment to maintain her strength, and the fetus was treated in utero at fourteen and twenty-six weeks to ensure that it had good digestion, was strong, and had plenty of hair. She took zinc throughout and gave birth to a boy without difficulty. She also found that using lavender and neroli essential oils in an oil base prevented stretch marks.

Cranial Osteopathy

By working through the bones of your head, a cranial osteopath can affect the action of the pea-sized pituitary gland, which governs the output of hormones. This can be particularly useful for women whose periods are irregular or who are not ovulating.

Some cranial osteopaths work directly on the organs through the abdomen, which can free adhesions and get the uterus working normally.

Sharon had not become pregnant although she and her husband had been trying for two years. She had cranial treatment to improve the function of her pituitary gland and get her hormones functioning better and work on her pelvis to improve the drainage from the uterus and improve the blood supply to the ovaries. Within two months she was pregnant and went on to have a healthy boy. Three years later she had not managed to conceive again and further treatment eventually resulted in her having a daughter. She subsequently became pregnant without treatment.

Herbal Medicine

It is best to consult a practitioner for an individual diagnosis, although there are herbs that you can try on your own. Red clover flowers are thought to be an effective tonic for women. Combine one ounce (25 g) of flowers with a teaspoon (5 ml) of peppermint and infuse in two pints (1.2 liters) of water; drink it freely throughout the day. Nettle *(Urtica dioica)* tea and raspberry leaf tea should also be taken daily, at least a cupful each day. False unicorn root *(Chamaelireum luteum)* is good for correcting hormonal imbalances and can be taken as a tincture, five to fifteen drops daily. The berries of the chaste tree, *Vitex agnus castus*, have an unrivaled reputation for their ability to affect the pituitary gland and normalize estrogen and progesterone output. Try taking ten to twenty drops of *Vitex agnus castus* three times a day. For ovarian dysfunction, try vitex and false unicorn root (simmer one to two teaspoons of root in a cup of water for ten to fifteen minutes then drink as tea).

Men should try oats (can be eaten as hot cereal or as a fluid extract, thirty to forty drops three times per day) and sarsaparilla (ten to fifteen drops three times per day).

Homeopathy

Homeopathy can work well in cases of infertility. Treatment must be from a professional homeopath.

Hypnotherapy

It can be hard to accept that fertility can be affected by the mind and that for some unconscious reason you are not allowing pregnancy to take place, even harder perhaps that your subconscious can maintain this hold even when you are asleep. However, everyone knows of at least one person who was unable to conceive and yet became pregnant once adoption proceedings were started or was told that nothing more could be done medically and then conceived without any assistance at all. Hypnotherapy can, on occasion, deal with the matters that trouble both men and women subconsciously so that the blocks that prevent conception are removed.

Reflexology

Reflexology has a good reputation for curing infertility, partly by reducing stress levels. It is recommended that both partners be treated in cases of unexplained infertility.

Melanie had been trying to become pregnant for three and a half years. She started reflexology treatment and had an hour's work on her feet once a week for six months and then fortnightly for a further three months. As treatment progressed, she could feel a change in her feet and found that she became more aware of her body and less hyped-up about not becoming pregnant. She enjoyed the feeling of being pampered and the opportunity to talk to the reflexologist, who listened without being judgmental.

She also asked for a referral to a gynecologist, but by the time the appointment arrived, fourteen months after she started the reflexology, she was four months pregnant. She went on to have a healthy baby girl.

5

Conception

It might seem as though conception is the easy part—after all, you have probably been practicing for years. However, having made the decision to have a baby, you will find it useful to know when to try. Each month there is only a surprisingly short time during which a woman is fertile. This information becomes useful later to avoid pregnancy.

THE FERTILITY CYCLE

Ovulation, the release of an egg from the ovary, ripe for fertilization, takes place roughly fourteen days before a period starts. This means it is midway through a twenty-eight-day cycle, but could be a week later, i.e., twenty-one days after the start of a period for someone with a thirty-five-day cycle. If you have regular cycles, timing conception should be relatively easy, but if you do not, there are other ways of working out when ovulation is taking place.

Conception takes place when a sperm meets and fertilizes an egg or ovum, after it has been released from the ovary where it has been ripening. The egg develops in a follicle on the ovary; boosted by hormones, the follicle eventually bursts and discharges the egg (occasionally two) into the pelvic cavity, where it is scooped up by the mobile fringe of one of the fallopian tubes and is wafted down the tube toward the uterus. Although sperm can survive for three to five days, the egg lives for only twelve to twenty-four hours, so that for fertilization to take place, intercourse should have occurred either within the two or three days prior to ovulation or within the few hours after it. Considering the circumstances, it seems astonishing that overpopulation could ever be a problem.

CHARTING OVULATION

Ovulation can be determined by taking your temperature daily, by being aware of the changes in cervical mucus, and possibly by individual body signs. There are also a couple of commercial tests available.

Even if you do not know when you ovulate, you may be aware that the type of mucus discharge from your vagina changes in quality and quantity throughout the month. With practice you can become familiar with the different types and recognize the kind that indicates you are about to ovulate. It may be easiest to start by directly feeling your cervix every day. The best way to do this is by washing your hands, leaving them wet, and then squatting or sitting on the toilet. Insert one or two fingers into your vagina as far as they will go. The cervix, the base of the uterus located at the top of your vagina, will feel like a firm smooth knob with a little indentation in the middle, which is the os or opening to the uterus. The uterus is attached in the pelvis by ligaments so that it is slightly mobile, and its position in relation to the vagina alters during the month. At the start of the cycle the cervix is low, rising two to three centimeters at ovulation to its highest point, when it is hardest to reach with your fingers, and then becoming low in the vagina again as your period approaches. At ovulation the os opens slightly and the vagina becomes softer and more accommodating.

The most striking difference, however, is in the amount and texture of the mucus coming from the cervix during the course of the menstrual cycle. Mucus that follows a period is fairly scanty, sticky, dry, opaque, and pastelike. As the time of ovulation approaches, the mucus becomes much wetter and more slippery. It also becomes clearer, more profuse, and stretchy enough to string it between two fingers; it has a consistency not unlike egg white at this time. There may be sufficient quantities of mucus to make your underpants feel wet. This change in mucus occurs at ovulation in order to enable the sperm to swim rapidly through it and up the cervical canal. Under ideal conditions sperm can reach the fallopian tubes in five minutes.

Once ovulation has taken place, indicated by a peak day with the maximum mucus loss, the cervix and mucus return quite rapidly to their preovulatory state, when the cervix is low and hard, the os is closed, and the mucus is cloudier, stickier, and less plentiful. If you are using your fertility awareness as a method of contraception, you should be safe following the third day after the peak day.

You can also tell when you are ovulating by a method known as basal body temperature (BBT) charting. This involves using a special thermometer to take your temperature daily, either first thing in the morning before rising or at another set time, provided in both instances that you have nothing to eat or drink for an hour beforehand. Buy a fertility (basal) thermometer from a pharmacy, and using graph paper plot a chart with the days of the month along one axis and the possible range of temperatures along the other. It may be between 96.8°F (36.0°C) and 98.6°F (37.0°C) but depends on individual variation. Take your temperature, and then plot the result on the graph (this can be done later in the day if more convenient). At the end of your cycle, join the dots and you should have a chart with consistently lower readings in the first half of the cycle than in the second. In between the levels there should be a slight drop followed within a day or two by a noticeable rise of one-tenth of a degree Fahrenheit (0.2°C to 0.5°C). This indicates that ovulation has taken place. Charts are not always easy to interpret and can be affected by illness, so they are best used in conjunction with the other signs.

Other ways of anticipating ovulation include observing various body changes such as insomnia, tiredness, increased sex drive, fullness and tenderness of the breasts, vaginal odor, blemishes, or greasiness of hair. You might also feel cramplike pains on the right or left side of the body depending on which ovary has released the egg, vulval pressure, pains in the legs, nettle-rash, or other symptoms specific to you. Careful observation of your cycle will mean that you become well aware of your fertility and so are able to pick the right time to attempt conception.

Commercial tests, available from a pharmacy, can be used to detect the surge in luteinizing hormone indicating that ovulation is going to take place within the next twelve to twenty-four hours. They are expensive, but claim accuracy of prediction of around 66 percent for the first month of testing, increasing to 85 percent if used for longer. They can prove if you are failing to ovulate at all.

Timing Sexual Intercourse

In order to give yourself the best opportunity of becoming pregnant, have sex every other day from the day your cervical mucus starts to become wet until you are sure you have ovulated. You need only have sex once at ovulation—sex more frequently than every forty-eight hours can deplete the level of sperm. Make love in the conventional position, with a pillow under your bottom. Your partner should wait until his penis is limp before withdrawing, and you should stay on your back for half an hour. Be sure to make a note of the day in your diary.

Choosing the Sex of Your Child

Having sex around the time of ovulation should result in pregnancy, but you may particularly want a boy or girl. You can alter the odds so that you have an 80 to 85 percent chance of having a baby of the sex you want. In order to do this, you need to be as sure as possible of your time of ovulation and plan sex carefully around that time.

For a Boy

Abstain from sex for at least four days before ovulation; then have sex as close as possible to the moment of ovulation. Before intercourse, douche with a water and sodium bicarbonate solution in a dilution of one tablespoon (15 ml) to a pint (600 ml) of water. This produces the alkaline conditions that favor male (Y) sperm. Alkaline mucus is also produced by orgasm and this, together with full penetration at ejaculation, also helps.

For a Girl

Deliberately conceiving a girl is less easy because it requires anticipating the time of ovulation and having sex two or three days beforehand. You must then abstain until three days after ovulation. The douche for conceiving a girl is one tablespoon (15 ml) of white vinegar to a pint (600 ml) of water. The theory is that female sperm outlive male ones, and so they are the ones still in the fallopian tubes when the egg is released. The X sperm travel most easily in acid conditions.

THE FIRST SYMPTOMS OF PREGNANCY

Most women who have been pregnant once have a pretty good idea when they have conceived on subsequent occasions. The first time it is not as easy to be certain, but now you can get a result from a home pregnancy test the day that your period is due.

The fertilized egg travels down the fallopian tube, taking about five to seven days to reach the uterus. Once there the multiplying cells burrow into the endometrium, the lining of the uterus. This implantation site is the one where the placenta will develop. Some women actually feel implantation as strong contractions lasting several hours. Occasionally, there is a very slight blood loss.

From this time onward you may feel some of the symptoms of early pregnancy. Your breasts may feel tender or throb or tingle. They may swell and itch, or you might feel shooting pains in them. You may also be much thirstier and hungrier than usual, and as a result you may need to urinate more frequently. You might feel dizzy or unusually warm.

You will probably feel devastatingly tired and be ready to go to bed in the early evening, if not before. Often your digestion is completely upset, and you may have feelings of nausea or actually be sick. Some food and drink may completely lose its appeal, typically fatty food, coffee, and alcohol, and you may have cravings for some foods you don't normally like. Your sense of smell can be upset too; some smells can become nauseating and you can be haunted by unpleasant smells that no one else can smell. You may also have a metallic taste in your mouth.

If you have all these symptoms, you are almost certainly pregnant, but there are two other ways of telling. One is by means of your cervix. If your are pregnant, your cervix remains high and grows increasingly soft instead of becoming lower and hard as it usually does before a period. At the same time your vagina gradually changes color from its usual pink to a dusky purple-blue. You are also likely to be pregnant if your temperature stays high at the end of your cycle and does not drop just before the period is due, as it would normally. A temperature above 98.9°F (37.2°C) suggests pregnancy.

6

Preparing Yourself for Pregnancy and Birth

DIET

A healthy diet is of vital importance to the pregnant and lactating woman and to her growing baby. The baby is totally dependent on the mother for all nutrients, and it seems obvious he or she should be getting only the best. Moreover, well-nourished women tend to do much better in labor and their babies are born in better condition and are more healthy overall. There are two situations when it is easy to overlook this wisdom. If you suffer from morning sickness, it can be difficult to keep anything at all down and almost any healthy food can seem quite repulsive. The other is when you have been pregnant for some months, it seems most unlikely that you will ever be anything else and therefore no point in being careful about what you eat.

Ideally, you will be eating well before you conceive, but if not you should take time to work out a good diet once you are pregnant and able to tolerate a wide range of foods.

It is important to avoid the candy bar and cup of coffee syndrome even when very rushed. If this is your first baby, it can be difficult to modify your behavior because it is much harder to visualize the baby and be protective toward him or her. Your needs are all too obvious, whereas the baby's have to be guessed at. A good diet will help you feel better too and more able to cope with the demands pregnancy makes on your system.

Try to make sure that you eat at least three times a day. As you grow and there is less room in your stomach, it is often better to eat six small meals daily. Some general rules include the following:

- Avoid refined carbohydrates, making sure that most of your calories come from whole grains, potatoes, beans, and pulses.
- Eat plenty of fresh fruit and vegetables, at least some of them raw.
- Eat two to three ounces (60 to 80 g) of protein daily. Choose from meat, fish, eggs, milk, and dairy products.
- Eat dried fruit and nuts for snacks.
- Drink plenty of spring water.
- Avoid tea and coffee.

Nutritional Supplementation

Nutritional supplementation during pregnancy is a controversial issue. You may feel all nutrients are best obtained from eating well and that taking vitamins and minerals is potentially risky. On the other hand, you may feel that the baby's needs put a strain on your resources, which for various reasons such as poor health, poor diet, stress, or exhaustion are not at their best, and that as a result you want to provide the best for both of you by taking extra supplements. Some are suggested in the following pages.

Vitamin supplements taken prior to conception and during pregnancy have been shown to reduce the numbers of babies born with spina bifida to mothers who have previously had affected babies and whose subsequent children were at increased risk of being born with the condition. A study of more than 4,000 Hungarian women given a multivitamin tablet (including folic acid) for at least one month before and two months after conception showed a significant reduction in the incidence of other congenital abnormalities too.[1] See Table 1. A larger study has shown that taking calcium (2 g) as a supplement from the twelfth week of pregnancy can significantly lower the risk of having high blood pressure in later pregnancy.[2]

Table 1
CZEIZEL'S VITAMIN SUPPLEMENT CONTENTS

Vitamin A	6,000 I.U.
Vitamin B_1	1.6 mg
Vitamin B_2	1.8 mg
Vitamin B_6	2.6 mg
Vitmain B_{12}	4.0 mcg
Vitamin C	100 mcg
Vitamin D	500 I.U.
Vitamin E	15 mg
Nicorthamide	19 mg
Ca.-Pantothenate	10 mg
Biotin	0.2 mg
Folic Acid	0.8 mg
Calcium	125 mg
Phosphorus	125 mg
Magnesium	100 mg
Iron	60 mg
Copper	1 mg
Manganese	1 mg
Zinc	7.5 mg

Zinc deficiency seems to be a common finding in nonpregnant women and it is one of the things, together with folic acid, vitamin B, vitamin C, calcium, and magnesium, for which there is a 30 to 100 percent increase in need during pregnancy. Your diet has to be exceptionally good to meet these requirements. My research shows that zinc deficiency, more common in vegetarians, vegans, and those who have been anorexic, can be responsible for severe pregnancy sickness. If you wish to take supplements, a recommended regimen includes:

multivitamin
vitamin B complex
1 g vitamin C
calcium
magnesium
15 mg zinc

Vegans and vegetarians are advised to make sure they include three to four micrograms of vitamin B_{12} daily in their diets, even if they do not take the other supplements.

One note of warning here, no pregnant woman should take more than 5,000 I.U.s of vitamin A per day because high amounts can cause birth defects.[3] Liver and fish liver oils are high in vitamin A.

Natural Ways of Obtaining Vitamins and Minerals

The following list shows which vitamins and minerals can be found in specific foods.

Vitamin A—green, yellow, or orange vegetables; margarine; orange and yellow fruits; alfalfa; watercress; parsley; nettles; raspberry leaves.

Vitamin B Complex—whole grains, pork, beef, liver, beans, cereals, brown rice, milk, dairy products, eggs, bananas, avocados, nuts, seeds.

Vitamin B_6—meat, fish, egg yolk, whole grains, bananas, avocados, seeds, nuts.

Vitamin B_{12}—liver and other internal organs, meat, fish, dairy products, eggs, brewer's yeast, alfalfa, miso, seaweed.

Vitamin C—most fruits, green vegetables, liver, kidney, potatoes, elderberries, rosehips.

Vitamin D—fatty fish, cod liver oil, eggs, milk, butter, margarine, cheese, alfalfa, nettles, sunshine.

Vitamin E—vegetable oils, nuts, seeds, soy, lettuce, eggs, watercress, alfalfa, rosehips, raspberry leaves, dandelion, seaweed.

Vitamin K—turnips, greens, broccoli, cabbage, lettuce, liver, green tea, cereals, alfalfa, nettles, kelp.

Amino Acids (including lysine and arginine)—found in all first-class protein such as meat, fish, eggs, and dairy products.

Calcium—milk, cheese, broccoli, green leafy vegetables, nuts, seeds, peas, beans, lentils, alfalfa, red clover, raspberry leaves, nettles, parsley, watercress.

Chromium—brewer's yeast, whole grains, liver, cheese, molasses.

Copper—oysters, kidney, liver, dried peas and beans, nuts, spinach, cabbage, watercress, alfalfa, parsley, kale, nettles, chickweed.

Fluorine—spinach, watercress, garlic.

Folic Acid—liver, kidney, green vegetables, eggs, wholegrain cereals.

Iodine—shrimp, fish, beef liver, pineapple, eggs, peanuts, wholewheat bread, raisins, watercress, parsley, sarsaparilla, seaweed.

Iron—liver, kidney, heart, egg yolk, peas, beans, cocoa, molasses, shellfish, parsley, nettles, dandelion, alfalfa, yellow dock.

Magnesium—nuts, periwinkles and snails, shrimp, soy, whole grains, green leafy vegetables, tap water in hard water areas, watercress, alfalfa, parsley, carrot tops.

Manganese—green leafy vegetables, whole grains, spinach, alfalfa, parsley, watercress.

Phosphorus—milk and dairy products, nuts, whole grains, cereals, poultry, eggs, meat and fish, caraway seeds, parsley, watercress, nettles, chickweed, alfalfa, licorice, marigold petals, raspberry leaves.

Potassium—fresh fruits, vegetables, whole grains, chamomile, dandelion, parsley.

Selenium—eggs, fish, whole grains, brown rice, meat, poultry, nuts.

Silicon—spinach, horsetail, dandelion, nettles, leeks.

Sodium—salt, milk, cheese.

Sulfur—cabbage family vegetables, nettles, plantain, garlic.

Zinc—oysters, lamb chops, steak, pecans, split peas, brazil nuts, beef liver, nonfat dried milk, egg yolk, whole wheat, rye, oats, peanuts, watercress.

Supplements to Prepare for Labor

Some of the remedies designed to ease labor have to be taken during pregnancy. Raspberry leaf tea (or tablets), possibly combined with squaw vine *(Mitchella repens)*, is one such remedy. The tea can be taken once a day throughout pregnancy or three times a day for the last three months. It is rich in iron and vitamin C and aids digestion. It tones the uterus and helps to prevent hemorrhage. There are also various other prenatal tonics available from reputable herbalists.

The homeopathic equivalent is Caulophyllum, recommended as a prophylactic against a difficult labor. However, it is now felt that, as with any homeopathic remedy, it can be counterproductive to take it routinely or when there is no indicated need. It can in fact cause the symptoms that you are trying to avoid, in this case slow inefficient contractions, and can slow or stop labor and may result in bleeding. It does have a place if you are under threat of induction, or if your water has broken and contractions have not started. If it fails to start labor under these circumstances, consult a homeopath.

EXERCISE

Most women want to give birth as easily as possible, and there are a number of ways of preparing for the birth that should ensure that you are fit for the event. Exercise is one of the ways of getting in training. You can enroll in a yoga class specifically for pregnant women, and there are many other types of prenatal exercise classes available. If you cannot reach a class, you can follow your own exercise routine at home. A good program is described in *New Life* by Janet and Arthur Balaskas, for example.

Swimming and cycling are particularly helpful forms of exercise. Swimming uses every muscle in your body, and the water supports your weight, something that becomes increasingly welcome as pregnancy progresses. Cycling too takes your weight while you get fitter, and it can also help to widen your pelvic outlet.

Two important exercises that should be practiced daily are the pelvic floor exercise and squatting. You should be able to spend as long as fifteen minutes in an unsupported squat by the end of pregnancy, although for various reasons not everyone manages this. When you first start, you may find that you need the support of a wall and need to put a couple of books under your heels. However, if you practice squatting every day, you will eventually be able to squat unsupported with your heels flat on the floor, your back straight, and your knees apart. If you clasp your hands together under your chin, you can use your elbows to separate your knees.

The pelvic floor exercise (also called Kegel exercises) is useful for toning up the muscles around your perineum and learning to control those muscles so that you are able to relax them consciously at the moment of crowning. It is especially important to do the pelvic floor exercise after the birth to help tone up the pelvic muscles. Doing the exercise daily should reduce the risk of uterine prolapse in later life.

To do the exercise, first identify the muscles by trying to stop yourself in midflow of urine. These are the muscles you need to exercise. Practice contracting them slowly, holding them at their tightest for several seconds, and then slowly letting go. Try doing five at a time, several times a day.

Your capacity for exercise decreases as you get closer to the birth, but it is important to maintain some kind of activity because labor requires a lot of strength and energy, and the fitter you are the easier it is to cope.

PERINEAL MASSAGE

Massaging your perineum from about thirty weeks of pregnancy can help make it more supple and stretchy, so that it is better able to slide over the baby's head, rather than tearing, during the birth. Massage can also help to soften previous episiotomy scars.

The best time to start the massage is after a warm bath. Using an oil such as almond, olive, vitamin E, or wheatgerm or a nonpetroleum-based calendula ointment, lubricate your fingers. Then very gently insert two fingers into your vagina and gradually increase the space between them so that the skin becomes stretched, a bit like pulling out the corners of your mouth. You will find that as time goes by you will be able to accommodate more of your fingers. Hook your thumb into your vagina and pull the perineum outward, massaging the skin with the oil in a U-shape while concentrating on any area of tenderness or previous scarring. You will find that the whole area softens as you get closer to delivery, but massaging daily can make a real difference to your perineum.

Prenatal Classes

Prenatal classes may provide an opportunity for you to discuss particular anxieties and share the experience of becoming parents with others at a similar stage. As in all self-help groups, the members will provide a special understanding that can only be obtained from those who are feeling just the way you are at present.

Birth Attendants

One way of making your birth easier is to have someone with you, as well as or instead of the baby's father. This might be someone who has had children herself, knows intuitively how you are feeling and how you can be helped, and feels the excitement and privilege of being at a birth. Although it is not customary at present, evidence from a large study in the United States shows that the presence of doulas—lay birth companions—has a very positive effect in terms of outcome and duration of labor. It can be enormously helpful to have a sympathetic person with you, someone who has been through it herself, to provide additional support and comfort. If you do not know anyone to ask, you could try asking your prenatal teacher to attend your birth—many would be thrilled to be asked. If you are planning a hospital birth, make sure well in advance that you will be able to have the people of your choice with you. Some hospitals have policies limiting you to one partner only, but this is subject to negotiation.

REBIRTHING

One way of preparing yourself for childbirth, rebirthing is a simple breathing technique based on the principle that there is a direct connection between physical and mental well-being and that breathing is the key element in liberating the body from tension, fear, and pain. It can help you to become more in touch with your feelings and allows you to recognize and release hurtful memories.

An A~Z of Possible Problems and Their Remedies

ANEMIA

A sample of your blood will be taken several times during your pregnancy to test, among other things, for the hemoglobin level. Hemoglobin (Hb) is a measure of the quantity and quality of the red oxygen-carrying cells in your body. The scale ranges from 14.7 g downward, and you are considered anemic if your Hb is 11 g or lower. Anemia is more likely to occur in the last three months or so of pregnancy when the baby's need for iron is greatest. Anemia can make you feel very tired and deplete your reserves so that blood loss at delivery could be serious, which is why women are often given iron and folic acid supplements. However, the value of routine supplementation is being questioned, in part because only 7 percent of pregnant women suffer from anemia anyway. In addition, high levels of iron are thought to predispose a woman toward postpartum hemorrhage and may make the red cells so large that they are unable to cross the placenta. Iron supplements can also cause jet-black stools, constipation, hemorrhoids, and nausea.

The best way to avoid the need for iron tablets is to make sure that you include plenty of iron-rich foods in your diet. Good sources of iron include lean meat (especially kidney), wheatgerm, egg yolk, watercress, dried fruit, celeriac, butter beans, kidney beans, dark green vegetables, cream, cottage cheese, and cocoa.

If you know you are anemic, you could try taking an herbal preparation rich in iron. Iron is better assimilated by the body if it is taken along with vitamin C. Certain foods such as bran, tea, and coffee can actually inhibit the body's ability to absorb iron from food and should be avoided if possible. Drinking tea at mealtimes seems to be the most harmful.

It is quite possible that you may not need any supplementation if you are eating a properly balanced diet. Moreover, you may be clinically anemic and yet feel fine. It is thought by some people that some degree of anemia is normal during pregnancy because of the great increase in blood volume. The hemoglobin returns to normal after delivery, when a lot of excess fluid is shed.

If you are tired but not anemic, you may be helped by taking oil of evening primrose (1 to 3 g).

Acupuncture

You can be treated successfully by acupuncture so it is worth seeking advice from a specialist.

Homeopathy

It is best to consult a homeopath for an individual diagnosis, although Ferrum or Ferrum magneticum 9x potency helps anemia in many women. Ask your pharmacist about suitable iron preparations that are released gradually into the body. Let her or him know how many months pregnant you are; large doses of iron are not recommended during the first trimester.

BACKACHE

Backache can seem an inevitable part of pregnancy. It occurs as a consequence of the softening effect the hormone relaxin has on your ligaments in preparation for giving birth and as a result of carrying the weight of the growing baby at the front of your body. The additional weight tends to make you thrust your shoulders back and your stomach forward in order to maintain your balance, and this invariably puts a strain on your spine.

It is easier to prevent backache than it is to cure it once it has started. You can help yourself by maintaining the strength of your back through exercising. Such exercises are best started before pregnancy, but they will help even if you are already suffering from backache. Swimming is the best form of exercise, and yoga is very helpful too.

The other method of prevention is to pay careful attention to your posture. Try to think about balancing the baby in your pelvis like an egg in an egg cup. Do this by flattening the curve of your back and bending your knees slightly when standing. It is not always easy to remember to do this, but you can get into the habit of it if you practice for a while. It is particularly important to adopt this posture if you are standing for any length of time.

Shoes with even a slight heel can put an extra strain on your back, so it is best to wear flat-heeled shoes throughout pregnancy. It will also help to sit upright on a hard chair rather than slouching on a sofa and to sleep on a reasonably hard mattress. Put boards underneath your mattress if it is too soft.

Some women are helped by wearing a maternity girdle available in specialist corsetry shops or department stores. It may also help to take a calcium supplement (2 g from twelfth week of pregnancy). Remember that vomiting while bending over the toilet or basin can damage your spine. Problems in your dorsal spine can irritate the vagus nerve leading to the stomach and lead to further vomiting, resulting in a vicious circle of illness. See also information about sacroiliac joint pain on page 85.

Homeopathy

If your spine or sacrum or hips feel weak and you feel worse for stooping and walking, take Aesculus. If you feel exhausted and have a burning in the spine and the small of your back feels weak (it is worse in

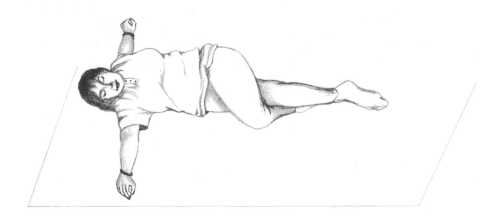

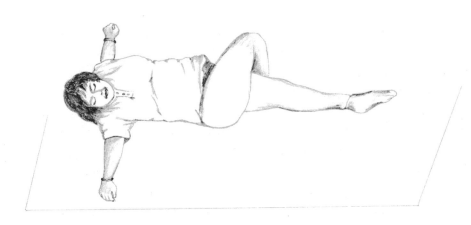

Exercise to relieve backache. The following hip rotation exercise helps relieve backache. Lie flat on your back and stretch your arms out to the side. Keep one leg straight and hook the foot of the other under your calf. Keeping your shoulders on the ground, twist your hips so that the knee of the bent leg touches the ground as nearly as possible. Hold for a few seconds and then repeat the exercise using the alternate leg. Also try crawling on all fours, keeping your spine straight and your pelvis tucked under you. Exercises taught in yoga or prenatal exercise classes will help too.

cold weather and on lying on your left and better with warmth and motion), take Kali. carb.

Take Arnica every three hours if backache is due to overexertion. For lameness due to the pressure of the baby take Bellis perennis.

Osteopathy

For persistent backache that is not relieved by any of these measures, see an osteopath or chiropractor for an individual diagnosis and treatment.

Reflexology

Reflexology can treat lower back pain and sacroiliac joint pain.

BLEEDING IN PREGNANCY

Slight bleeding in pregnancy does not necessarily mean that the fetus is at risk. Although it is not common, it does occur in around 10 percent of pregnancies up to twenty-eight weeks and slightly fewer after that time. It may be experienced as a slight loss at the time of the expected period and sometimes at fourteen weeks when the placenta takes over hormone production from the corpus luteum (a yellow body that grows on the ovary in place of the ruptured follicle and sustains the pregnancy until this point). It can also be caused by cervical polyps and erosions; these often bleed after intercourse, which is disconcerting but has no effect on the pregnancy. They can be seen with the aid of a speculum.

Less common, but potentially dangerous, is bleeding from an ectopic pregnancy. This is when the pregnancy establishes itself somewhere other than in the uterus, generally in one of the fallopian tubes. Bleeding starts sometime between six and twelve weeks and may be accompanied by one-sided abdominal pain. The growing embryo eventually distends the tube until it ruptures, causing pain, shock, and bleeding both internally and from the vagina. Surgery is required urgently in these circumstances in order to terminate the pregnancy and repair or remove the tube.

Bleeding after twenty-eight weeks can be caused by the placenta peeling away from the uterine wall before delivery. It will be accompanied by continuous pain and shock, because the blood loss is internal too. This is an indication for immediate medical attention because the baby is being deprived of oxygen, and the mother's life is also at risk. If abruptio placenta, as it is known, is diagnosed, the baby must be delivered by emergency cesarean section.

Another cause of bleeding in later pregnancy is placenta previa, which is caused by the placenta developing in the lower part of the uterus so that it totally or partially blocks the cervix. Once the cervix starts to stretch in preparation for labor, the placenta can be torn from its site and painless, bright red bleeding takes place. Placenta previa can be detected by ultrasound. If it is, a woman may be expected to spend the last months of pregnancy in a hospital because the risk of a sudden, disastrous hemorrhage is high, and the baby must be delivered by cesarean section. If the placenta only partially blocks the cervix, normal delivery is possible, although it must take place in a hospital.

Bleeding can also occur normally at the start of labor, quite heavily in some cases. If it is heavy enough to soak a pad, you should contact your midwife, doctor, or hospital.

Homeopathy

There are some very specific treatments for bleeding in pregnancy, depending on the cause and character of the bleeding. There is a homeopathic remedy for marginal placenta previa—take Erigeron 3x three times a day until the problem is gone, perhaps three to four weeks. Everyone should take Arnica as soon as the bleeding starts.

Causes

- From trauma—Arnica and cinnamon. If there is a delay in getting the actual remedy, you can make a tea from ground cinnamon as a temporary substitute.
- From fright—Aconite. If the fright has turned to shock, a state of near paralysis or nonreaction, stupor, or even unconsciousness—Opium.
- From anger or temper, even if it is not yours—Chamomilla.
- From excitement, agitation, manic states—Cimicifuga.

- From mental depression, shock, strain caused by nursing the sick—Baptisia.
- From debility—Aletris farinosa; Caulophyllum; China; Helonias; Secale.
- If degeneration of the placenta is diagnosed—Phosphorus.

Character of blood

- Dark, fluid—Secale.
- Light, fluid—Millefolium.
- Hemorrhage that will not stop—Thlapsi bursa.
- Intermittent, with spasmodic pains, wants fresh air—Pulsatilla.
- Laborlike pains, no bleeding—Secale.
- Pains from the back, around the abdomen, and down thighs; crampy squeezing—Viburnum.
- Partly clotted, with pains from small of back to pubis, worse from motion—Sabina.
- With pains from small of back to thighs, weak back, worse from motion—Kali. carb.
- Scanty or long oozing, irregular pains with weakness and trembling—Caulophyllum.

BLEEDING GUMS

The softening action of progesterone can mean that your gums bleed every time you clean your teeth. Rinsing your mouth with a drop of any of the following essential oils in water can be useful in helping to prevent it and the sour taste it can leave behind: geranium, frankincense, lavender. (Be sure not to swallow the solution.)

BREECH BABY

A baby is said to be in a breech position if at birth, or before, it presents its bottom first rather than its head. The delivery of breech babies is becoming an increasingly contentious issue. Formerly, these children, 3 percent of all babies at full-term, were delivered at home by doctors or midwives experienced in breech deliveries. Nowadays, the skill is being lost, and in many cases breech presentation is an automatic indication for delivery by cesarean section. The concern about the breech position is that the baby's head may be subject to sudden pressure after the rapid delivery of the body and that there is only a limited amount of time in which to get the baby's head through the pelvis. If you want to try having your breech baby vaginally, you may have to search for an understanding obstetrician or independent midwife willing to help you. An upright, active birth without an epidural is the best way to birth a breech baby.

Needless to say, it is far more satisfactory to persuade the baby to turn so that it is head-down well before birth, and there are a number of ways of attempting this. In fact, the baby only starts to become fixed at around thirty-two weeks in a first pregnancy and at around thirty-four weeks in subsequent ones, so it is not worth worrying about its position before then, unless you have had a breech baby before. You may suspect your baby is breech if you can feel its hard round head under your ribs, and you can get a sudden feeling of urgency if the baby kicks you in the bladder. Once you are certain that it is the wrong way up, start by giving gravity a chance. The head is the heaviest part of the baby, and inverting yourself, ideally head down in a swimming pool for as long and as often as you can manage, should provide a good opportunity for a shift of position. You can practice a modified version of this exercise at home by lying with your hips much higher than your head—either on your back with a pile of cushions under your bottom and the soles of your feet on the floor or by kneeling on the floor with your bottom in the air and your head resting on your arms on the floor. Sleep on your back with three or four pillows under your bottom.

Try to relax completely and talk to the baby, telling it why you want it to move and visualizing it head down. If the baby's bottom has engaged, you will need to perform the exercise with a steeper angle. If the baby does turn late, you may feel it as a great and possibly painful churning in your abdomen. Don't give up hope; babies have been known to turn at forty weeks.

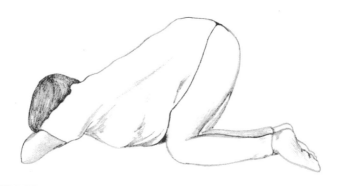

The knee-chest position. Kneel with your head on the floor with your bottom in the air and your head resting on your arms.

Acupuncture

Acupuncture has a good record of success in turning babies. The treatment should be started at thirty-five weeks, and you can either visit a practitioner or try the technique—known as moxibustion—at home. It involves the burning of moxa or mugwort, a slow-burning herb, over the skin beside the nail of both little toes. If you can get moxa, make a small cone of it and light it with a joss stick so that it smoulders rather than burns with a flame. If you cannot get moxa, you can hold a cigarette one-quarter inch (5 mm) away from the skin. Allow it to warm but not burn your skin for ten minutes on each little toe twice a day until the baby moves.

This treatment is useful for any malposition.

Homeopathy

Try Pulsatilla 200x in two doses, two days apart in the thirty-fifth week. Pulsatilla is also good for altering a baby's position in labor. Alternatively, consult a homeopath for an individual diagnosis and treatment.

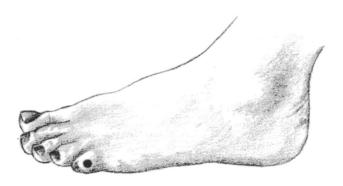

Acupressure point for turning malpositioned baby. Burn moxa or mugwort over the skin beside the nail of the little toes.

CONSTIPATION

This is a common complaint in pregnancy and occurs because the high levels of progesterone in the bloodstream act on the smooth muscles of the intestine to slow it down. You can improve the situation by altering your diet, exercising more, and changing your posture while sitting. For the latter, try sitting on a tilted chair—the kind that keeps your back straight, so that your knees are lower than your hips.

Dietary changes include eating more fruit, vegetables, nuts and seeds, and dried fruit. Bran is not necessarily helpful because it can reduce iron absorption. It will also help to eat fiber-rich foods, such as lentils, oats, and whole grains and to avoid refined carbohydrates. Red meat can cause constipation and should be replaced in the diet with fish and poultry.

Dehydration can result in constipation; in this case it might be accompanied by a headache. This will be improved by drinking several pints of spring water or diluted fruit juice daily.

Some of the other causes of constipation include taking iron tablets and drinking too much milk and tea. Try taking a liquid herbal iron supplement instead of iron tablets cutting down on dairy products, and drinking herbal teas.

Chewing gum helps some sufferers. Others may find that psyllium seeds (two teaspoonfuls in water) taken first thing in the morning improve matters. Nelson's hemorrhoid ointment can make it easier to pass stools even if you do not have hemorrhoids.

Acupuncture

Treatment provided by an acupuncturist can be very successful in dealing with the problem of constipation during pregnancy.

Herbal Medicine

Try drinking one cup of rhubarb root tea each night before going to bed. See remedies for hemorrhoids, pages 68–70.

Homeopathy

If your habits are sedentary and you have hard, dry stools, and an inactive rectum so that even soft stools are passed with difficulty, take Alumina. If you feel as though the bowel movement is incomplete and the condition is worse away from home, try Lycopodium. For fruitless, urging, obstinate constipation, in which you strain to pass a small amount and are irritable, take Nux vomica. For obstinate constipation, no urging for days, prolonged straining, and the feeling of a ball in the rectum, the remedy is Sepia.

For constipation associated with hemorrhoids that bleed and are painful, take Hydrastis.

If you are constipated and have a splitting headache and a dry mouth, feel thirsty, and are irritable and want to keep still, take Bryonia.

Massage

Lying on your back, try stroking with the fingers of both hands down the midline of your stomach from your chest to your pubic bone, up either side to your armpits, over your breasts, and down again. Repeat this twenty-one times.

Using mandarin or orange essential oil in the massage oil can help, although mandarin should be avoided in the first three to four months of pregnancy.

Nutritional Supplements

Taking magnesium daily (200 mg) can help, especially if you have suffered from premenstrual syndrome. Also try taking vitamin C (1 to 5 g per day).

Reflexology

A reflexologist can help improve constipation.

CRAMPING

Sudden sharp pains in the feet or legs can be an indication of cramping, a condition that is common in pregnancy. There are quite a few remedies, some for immediate use, others long-term.

When a cramp hits you, grab your toes and pull them toward your knees, or get out of bed and stand at arm's length from the wall, with your palms flat against it. Keeping your feet flat on the floor, lean toward the wall and stay in this position until the cramp is gone. Alternatively, you can pinch the area in between the root of your big toe and the one next to it, applying pressure firmly.

The other measures include getting up slowly in the morning, not stretching your legs fully, and doing eye-rolling exercises first (look out the corner of your eye to the furthest point possible to stretch your eye muscles, then slowly roll your eyes around to cover all directions). Elevating the head of your bed may help, or try wearing an anklet of corks or placing a cork under the mattress or pillow. Some find that eating a banana at bedtime works well also, if the cramping is due to a potassium deficiency.

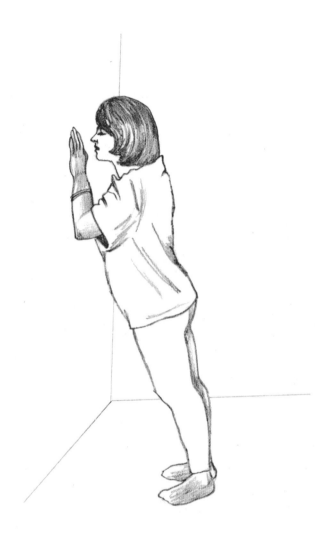

Muscle cramps in pregnancy. To relieve cramps in the feet or legs, stand at arm's length from the wall with your palms flat against it. Keeping your feet flat on the floor, lean toward the wall and stay in this position until the cramps are gone.

Aromatherapy

Hot foot baths with ten drops of lavender oil can be very beneficial, or take a bath in the evening before going to bed and massage your legs with oil to which a few drops of marjoram have been added.

Herbal Medicine

Two or three cups of hot cramp bark decoction daily may help.

Homeopathy

Crush three pills of Mag. phos. (standard 6x potency) with a little warm water and sip as needed.

Nutritional Supplements

Increase your calcium and magnesium intake to 210 and 130 mg, respectively, per day. Also, take a vitamin B-complex supplement that contains 50 mg B_6 daily. A teaspoonful of salt at tea-time can work wonders.

CYSTITIS

This unpleasant affliction can strike quite suddenly. It is caused by an inflammation of the bladder and results in a frequent and painful desire to urinate, even when the bladder is empty. Passing urine gives rise to a sensation of burning and stinging. It can be helped by drinking several pints of water, each containing one teaspoonful of sodium bicarbonate. If you start as soon as you feel the first twinge, a full-blown attack can be averted. The more you can drink the better.

Some people are particularly susceptible to cystitis and there is some evidence of a possible link with both candida (see pages 88–90) and food allergies (see page 173). If you suffer from cystitis frequently, you should see if either of these apply to you. For instance, a diet journal might indicate a link between your attacks and what you eat.

You can also take steps to prevent an attack of cystitis by not getting chilled, wearing cotton underclothes, and avoiding alcohol and sugary and spicy foods. Always urinate after making love. If home measures fail to clear up cystitis, it may be necessary to see your doctor for some antibiotics, because of the risk of kidney infection. If you do need to take antibiotics, make sure that you take lactobacillus capsules at the same time and eat plenty of live natural yogurt.

Aromatherapy

Try taking two drops of bergamot oil in a little alcohol.

Diet

A dietary regimen that can help is as follows:

Day 1 Drink at least four pints (2.25 l) of water with a teaspoonful of sodium bicarbonate per pint (500 ml) as above. Make a soup with barley and vegetables and drink lots of the strained liquid.

Day 2 Include brown rice and vegetables and fish in the diet.

Day 3 Gradually return to a normal diet, avoiding meat until there have been no symptoms for forty-eight hours.

Herbal Medicine

You can take hot yarrow tea every two hours. Yarrow can also be combined with equal parts of bearberry leaves and couch grass roots to help ease the symptoms. Or try a teaspoonful of powdered marshmallow root in a cupful of boiling water. This forms a paste that can be sweetened with honey and taken three times a day before meals. This should help lessen the distressing burning sensation experienced when urinating.

Homeopathy

Take Cantharis 6x three times a day for three days.

EDEMA (HEAVY SWELLING)

Some swelling of legs, hands, and feet is common during pregnancy. Excessive swelling, which is very uncomfortable, may be reduced by stimulation of the lymphatic drainage system. Try applying constant pressure to a point in the muscle above each breast on the side nearest your armpit. If you feel around, you should find a spot that is particularly tender. Simultaneously pressing and rubbing it will probably feel sore, but if done gently and daily can reduce fluid retention.

Nutritional Supplements

Vitamin B$_6$ taken as a 10-mg tablet daily has been shown to prevent edema from developing and may reduce it significantly if taken once it has become a problem.[1]

Edema sometimes leads to compression of a large nerve at the wrist. This results in pain and numbness in the fingers, and can lead to you dropping things. Vitamin B$_6$ (up to 200 mg daily) in a B-complex formula sometimes helps.

Reflexology

Reflexology is good at reducing the swelling caused by fluid retention in pregnancy.

FAINTING

This is common in early pregnancy, especially early in the morning or after a hot bath. It is due to progesterone acting on the smooth muscle and relaxing the muscles in the walls of your veins, with the result that blood pools in the legs and your brain becomes short of oxygen. The best remedy is to sit down with your head between your legs, and avoid rising suddenly if you are prone to faintness.

Dr. Bach's Rescue Remedy—a few drops in water or under the tongue—will help too.

Aromatherapy

Try a combination of eucalyptus, lemon, and lavender oils either in a bath, in a massage oil, or in a diffuser.

Homeopathy

For vertigo, with falling to the left or backward with a hot head, take Belladonna. With nausea, which is worse with traveling, being outside, or from emotions, take Cocculus. And for momentary loss of consciousness, which is worse outside or in the morning or after dinner and better with resting, the remedy is Nux vomica.

FATIGUE

Fatigue is closely allied with motherhood. It is an extremely common side effect of early pregnancy and many women spend the first trimester desperate for extra sleep. Toward the end of pregnancy, it is common to sleep poorly due to frequent need to urinate and difficulty in getting comfortable. This can seem like an unwelcome training program for the nights following the birth, when frequent night feeds will cause you to be more tired than you ever thought possible.

Unfortunately, the best remedy—more sleep—is often the one that is least available. At any stage it is a good idea to cut down on your activities whenever possible, so that you can sleep or rest more. This may mean that you need to make some radical changes in your lifestyle and perhaps accept that becoming a parent does make a difference to the way you live. In the early stages of pregnancy you may need to go out less or reduce your working hours; later on you may also need to nap during the day. If you are completely exhausted as a new mother, you should abandon everything that is not essential to survival. This can be particularly difficult because you may feel pressured to cope and also because you may feel that your individuality is being lost if all you can do is cater for the baby and yourself. Anemia can also cause fatigue (see pages 47–48).

Taking oil of evening primrose can help to counter the effects of fatigue. Try taking up to six 500-mg capsules a day.

Coffee, tea, chocolate, colas, and sweet foods can make tiredness worse by providing an instant energy boost that is followed by an energy low. Consequently, it is best to avoid such foods and drinks if you are feeling very tired.

FEARFULNESS AND TENSION

Fear of labor is normal, especially if you have not been through it before. It may not bother you too much; you may just feel a lurch in the stomach when you realize that one way or another the baby must come out. You can use this anxiety positively by making sure you feel comfortable about where you give birth, discussing it with your midwives and friends and at classes, making sure that you are fit for birth, eating well, and being well informed.

However, anxiety can mount so that fears about the birth come to dominate your life, giving you sleepless nights and wretched days. This may be from fear of the unknown or because you have some reason to think that there is something wrong with the baby or because you have had problems with this pregnancy or in previous ones. This type of anxiety can be all-consuming and is not constructive. If your concern cannot be used to alter and improve matters, then determine to either forget it or worry about it only between certain hours, say 9:00 and 10:00 A.M. Once you can do this, you may realize how even fretting for that length of time is fruitless.

Fear and tension during labor can slow the labor down and may result in unnecessary intervention. It can help to be very open about the way you are feeling—a good midwife or partner will be able to encourage and reassure you. Tension builds up not only as a result of pain but also because of the circumstances you may find yourself in, which is why it is important to have as much control of your situation as is possible. You may be taught conscious relaxation techniques in prenatal classes, and it is useful to use these to eliminate tension as far as possible.

Acupuncture

Acupuncture can improve prenatal depression.

Aromatherapy

Essential oils that lift the spirits are jasmine, clary sage, or ylang ylang. Put a few drops in your bath or float some in a saucer of warm water and inhale the aroma.

Homeopathy

For feelings of sudden fear, take Aconite. For a sensation of nervousness, take the tissue salt, Kali. phos. If you find yourself weeping frequently for no apparent reason, take Pulsatilla.

Hypnotherapy

You might also be helped by hypnotherapy, which can not only remove the anxiety but also can teach you techniques for pain relief during labor.

Technique for Relaxing

Find a comfortable position, in which you will be warm and free from distractions. Starting with your toes and working upward, become aware of any tension in any part of your body and let it go. Focus on your feet, ankles, calves, thighs, pelvis, stomach, chest, shoulders, arms, hands, neck, face, jaw, mouth, and scalp in turn. When you first practice this technique, you may find it easier to relax if you first tense each of the muscles for ten seconds before letting go. Become aware of how those muscles feel when relaxed, and take three slow breaths before you move on to the next group of muscles.

As you become more relaxed you will feel warmer, softer, and heavier. If extraneous thoughts distract you, concentrate on pleasant images— imagine that you are lazing on a beach or in an idyllic garden or try to fill your whole mind with your favorite color. As you become good at relaxing in this way, you can start to practice it in the sort of upright position that is best for labor.

FORGETFULNESS

Pregnancy can have a temporary but devastating effect on your brain. Women speak of starting to talk and then forgetting completely what they were going to say, being unable to remember if they have started doing something, or not being able to recall the names of things. Although your faculties are not necessarily impaired, it does seem that the impact of pregnancy hormones can change your memory and personality, causing you to react quite differently from the way you would if you were not pregnant.

The homeopathic remedy Nux moschata may help, and you can try and be meticulous about making lists and keeping appointments, but the only real remedy is giving birth. It can still take a while after the baby is born before you really get your brain back.

HEADACHES

Unfortunately, headaches are not uncommon during pregnancy, especially in the first few weeks. If you cannot avoid using painkillers, acetaminophen is preferable to aspirin. There are, however, other very effective ways of easing a headache that do not involve taking drugs.

Acupuncture

Headache during pregnancy is seen as being caused by a deficiency in the body, and the site of the headache indicates the type of deficiency, e.g., a headache on the top of the head means a problem in the liver. All types of pregnancy headache are treatable by acupuncture. You may be able to treat yourself with acupressure; see Julian Kenyon's book *Acupressure Techniques.*

Aromatherapy

Rub a few drops of lavender oil onto your temples. For a headache with nausea, a drop of peppermint oil can be taken on a cube of sugar.

A compress can be made by soaking a cloth in a half-pint (300 ml) of water to which six drops each of lavender and peppermint oil have been added. Lie down, put the cloth over your forehead, and relax. Rest is the best cure whenever possible.

Herbal Medicine

Try poppyhead tea or an infusion of equal parts of balm, lavender, and meadowsweet. Another remedy is to drop two cloves into a cup of tea, and allow them to infuse before drinking.

Nutritional Supplements

Zinc (25 mg per day) can have a wonderful effect on "hangover" headaches that appear on waking.

Important: Headache, together with disturbance of vision, such as seeing flashing lights, raised blood pressure, and severe fluid retention, can be a symptom of pre-eclampsia, a disease of the second half of pregnancy that if left untreated can develop into toxemia, a life-threatening condition (see information about hypertension, pages 70–72). Contact medical help if you get a severe headache that cannot be relieved with painkillers.

Reflexology

Reflexology can treat migraine and headaches caused by stress.

HEARTBURN

Heartburn is caused by the action of progesterone relaxing the valve at the upper end of the stomach so that the acid contents of the stomach can pass back into the esophagus. The condition is made worse by the growing baby pushing your stomach upward. The problem is relieved by delivery, but if you suffer from the unpleasant burning sensation in the chest that is heartburn, you will want a remedy well before then.

Some general suggestions include avoiding fatty, spicy, and acid foods, and alcohol and coffee. The best advice is to eat frequent small meals, being sure to chew well and slowly. Also, avoid bending or lying flat; it may help to sleep propped up and perhaps put a brick under the head of the bedstead. It is best to avoid prescription or over-the-counter antacids because, although they work initially, the stomach tends to increase its acid output to try and conteract the alkalinity. They also contain a lot of aluminium hydroxide, which can interfere with the absorption of certain nutrients and harm the fetus. Milk, too, works well but can have a rebound effect and increase the acid reflux.

Aromatherapy

In *Aromatherapy for Women*, Maggie Tisserand recommends one drop of sandalwood oil on the tongue. She suggests a drop of peppermint or rose oil as an alternative (avoid a large intake of essential oils while pregnant).

Oils that can be used externally include coriander, lemongrass, ginger, or lavender. Try them in the bath or diffuser, or use them in a base for massaging the abdomen and middle back.

Herbal Remedies

To neutralize acid and soothe the stomach, mix one teaspoon of slippery elm bark powder with honey or hot water. Or drink aniseed or fennel tea as your daily beverage, and try infusions of peppermint, meadowsweet, or chamomile to remedy heartburn. Chewing blanched almonds, dried papaya, or even washed orange peel may help too.

Eating several sprays of coriander leaves as a salad often cures chronic indigestion, or try eating half a teaspoonful of seeds mixed with honey raw before meals.

Homeopathy

For heartburn and indigestion linked with thrush, take Nat. phos. 6x tissue salt. With more definite flatulence and distension, which is worse after eating, take Carbo veg. If you have indigestion that feels like a stone in your stomach and have bitter eructations, take Nux vomica. If you have heartburn and dyspepsia after meals and are not thirsty, and it is made much worse by eating fatty things, take Pulsatilla.

HEMORRHOIDS

Hemorrhoids are varicose veins around the anus and are caused by pressure on relaxed blood vessels. They usually start with irritation and itching inside the rectum and around the anal area. They become worse on straining and can eventually protrude. The condition can be very painful, and there is no entirely satisfactory solution. Unfortunately, hemorrhoids tend to get worse with subsequent pregnancies, but they usually clear up after the birth. Occasionally, however, they are not present until after the birth when they appear suddenly and make the postpartum period very uncomfortable.

If you think that you are at risk of having hemorrhoids, do try to avoid becoming constipated (see page 56) as the extra straining will exacerbate the problem. Use an ointment such as Nelson's Cream for Hemorrhoids available from health food stores or Anusol from a pharmacy to relieve the discomfort. Apply the cream after every bowel movement and at night. It comes with a special applicator for inserting the ointment into the rectum. Minimize straining by using a squatting position on the toilet. This can be done by stacking magazines either side of the toilet and resting your feet on them. Pelvic floor exercises, concentrating on tightening the muscles around the anus, may help.

Put your feet up as much as you can, and try to rest with your bottom higher than your head. Hemorrhoids that protrude can be pushed back very gently with a finger. It may help to soften them first by sitting in a bath.

If you have a tendency toward hemorrhoids, do not practice unsupported squatting; instead lie on your back with your legs up against the wall.

If hemorrhoids remain prolapsed or if one becomes thrombosed, you will need to seek medical help.

Aromatherapy

Cypress oil can shrink hemorrhoids. Put a few drops in sitz bath of warm water, and sit in it for as long as you are comfortable.

Herbal Medicine

Take garlic perles, one to six per day (the one-a-day strength). Insert a peeled clove of garlic into the rectum at night. An infusion of lesser celandine (*Ranunculus ficaria*) three times a day or horsechestnut lotion (one cup boiling water with one to two teaspoons fruit, infused for ten to fifteen minutes) may also help relieve the symptoms. Another possibility is to apply live yogurt to the hemorrhoids. Try a moist compress of silverweed *(Potentilla tormentilla)* made with the lukewarm liquid created by boiling one pint of water with one to two tablespoons of chopped silverweed, then letting it stand for twenty minutes.

Homeopathy

For hemorrhoids with a sore, raw feeling, take Hamamelis. For blind (internal) hemorrhoids with back pain and constipation, take Calc. fluor. If they come on suddenly and are acute, inflamed, and make you feel restless and are worse with warmth, take Aconite. If they give rise to a stinging pain and are worse with backache and lying down, take Belladonna. If they are itching, burning, and oozing, perhaps with obstinate constipation or painless diarrhea, the remedy is Sulphur. For very sore, protruding, bleeding, hot hemorrhoids that are better with cold water and cause a bearing down feeling in the rectum, take Aloe.

HERPES

If you suffer from herpes, include vitamin B_{12} (as a complex) with brewer's yeast in your diet. Use acidophilus capsules as pessaries and take them orally. Apply goldenseal *(Hydrastis canadensis)* tincture locally and use an ice cube locally at the first sign of an outbreak. It is best to consult a homeopath for constitutional treatment, but Hepar sulph. 30x and Variolinum 30x once daily until there is an improvement should help.

HYPERTENSION (HIGH BLOOD PRESSURE)

Technically hypertension exists when the diastolic pressure has risen twenty or more points above your normal pregnancy blood pressure, i.e., if your blood pressure in early pregnancy was 120/70, then it is unsatisfactorily high if it reaches 140/90. The normal range in pregnancy is from 90/50 to 130/80. The upper figure—the systolic—denotes the pressure generated by your heart as it pumps blood around your body. The lower pressure—the diastolic—indicates the pressure in your arteries when the heart is at rest. This is the figure of most significance because a large increase in diastolic pressure means a reduction in the supply of blood and oxygen to the baby and indicates a risk of developing pre-eclampsia.

Pre-eclampsia, which can become toxemia, is a disease exclusive to the second half of pregnancy. Its cause is not fully known, although it is thought to be immunological. It is experienced by 12 percent of first-time mothers and only 4 percent of those having subsequent babies. If untreated it can lead to severe convulsions in the mother and the death of the baby. High blood pressure, protein in the urine, and excessive fluid retention constitute pre-eclampsia. It is a condition that can start quite suddenly, so the warning signs must be taken very seriously. These include:

- severe headaches that cannot be relieved by painkillers;
- visual disturbances, like seeing flashing lights;
- abdominal pain;
- considerable swelling.

If, however, your blood pressure is raised but you have no other signs of pre-eclampsia, you will probably want to find ways of reducing it. Otherwise you will be expected to rest while feeling perfectly fit. Moreover, high blood pressure is one of the indications for induction of labor.

Of course, eating well is important, although there are opposing theories about this. One, promoted by Dr. Tom Brewer, states that pre-eclampsia is a disease of malnutrition that can be prevented by eating a high-protein diet with salt to taste. Another maintains that blood pressure can be reduced by fasting on a diet of watermelon and brown rice; once it is back to normal, this theory suggests avoiding red meat, spicy foods, and alcohol and eating plenty of raw fruits and vegetables. Cut down on salt intake and drink six to eight glasses of pure spring water daily.

Acupuncture

Acupuncture can effectively reduce essential hypertension, i.e., chronically raised pressure that gives a high reading in early pregnancy. Acupuncture can also reduce blood pressure in women who have raised blood pressure close to full-term. This can be physically demonstrated with women whose blood pressure is so high that it is continuously monitored—a digital display shows blood pressure falling during treatment.

Herbal Medicine

Take garlic perles, between two and ten daily, or eat several cloves of raw garlic. Try drinking a dandelion infusion at least twice daily. You can also eat raw or cooked dandelion leaves as well. Take celery in any form, as stalks, juice, or seeds in celery salt or try celeriac. Overripe cucumber is said to be useful too. Alternatively, try one-quarter to one teaspoonful cayenne three times a day taken in orange juice or yogurt to normalize blood pressure.

Homeopathy

Kali. chlor. is the remedy for hypertension although it is probably best to consult a homeopath.

Nutritional Supplements

Take a B-complex supplement that includes Vitamin B_6 (50 mg) daily. Also take calcium (210 mg) and magnesium (130 mg) daily.

INSOMNIA

This is very common in late pregnancy for a number of reasons: it may be hard to get comfortable in bed, you may have to urinate several times a night, or be disturbed by the baby kicking. If you usually sleep on your stomach, trying to fall asleep on your side can be miserable.

There are practical steps that you can take. Use extra pillows under your bulge or prop yourself up. Keep a bucket at the bedside to use as a chamberpot, or perhaps sleep in a more comfortable bed. Many couples find that neither gets much rest in a double bed at this stage. It can help to get up and go into another room or make a drink of honey and lemon.

Sometimes anxiety can prevent you from sleeping, either by stopping you from falling asleep or by causing you to wake in the night, perhaps after dreadfully vivid nightmares about the baby or labor. You may find that discussing your anxieties with friends, midwife, or childbirth instructor helps. Other worries can be tackled by taking an objective view of your problems and seeing how you would advise a friend in the same situation.

Practicing relaxation techniques, avoiding daytime naps, and exercising daily can give you a better night's sleep.

Acupuncture

Acupuncture can have a very beneficial effect on sleeplessness at any time.

Aromatherapy

Massage at bedtime is soothing and relaxing and can encourage a sound sleep. Try putting a drop of neroli oil or clary sage on the edge of your pillow or using them in a massage oil.

You can also try scenting the bedroom with a few drops of chamomile and lavender essential oils in a diffuser or with water in a spray bottle.

Herbal Medicine

Try infusions made from any of the following herbs: hops, passion flower, elderflower, Californian poppy *(Eschscholzia california)*, or valerian. You can also try using them in baths. To prepare an herbal bath, pour two pints (1.2 liters) of boiling water onto one or two handfuls of the herb. Allow it to stand for half an hour, strain, then pour into a hot bath. Avena sativa compound from Weleda works well. Take ten to twenty drops in water half an hour before bed.

Homeopathy

Nelson–Bach Noctura tablets, a combination remedy, can be very effective (these contain sixth potency of Kali. brom, Coffea, Passiflora, Avena sativa, Alfalfa, and Valeriana). Or try Cocculus when you have difficulty in getting back to sleep again or Coffea crud. when sleeplessness results from excitement or too much coffee or when pain is unsupportable and too many thoughts are filling your mind.

Reflexology

Try visiting a reflexologist if insomnia becomes a chronic problem.

METALLIC TASTE IN THE MOUTH

You may find that you are plagued by an ever-present unusual taste of metal in your mouth. It tends to be a symptom of early pregnancy.

Herbal Medicine

Herbal remedies include mouthwashes with fennel, rosemary, and thyme. Weleda makes one that contains extracts of myrrh and krameria, the Peruvian toothbrush plant.

Homeopathy

If it is a strong, slimy taste with a lot of saliva, try the homeopathic remedy Cuprum met. 6x. If it is sweetish with coppery saliva, try Merc. sol. 6x.

Nutritional Supplements

A nutritional supplement of zinc (25 mg per day, or 15 mg of elemental zinc) if you are not already taking it, should help.

MISCARRIAGE

As many as one in two pregnancies fail to go full-term. The majority of those lost are in the very earliest stages of pregnancy, perhaps even before the first period is missed or in the days afterward. Women often suspect this when they experience symptoms of pregnancy and then have a late period, one which might be particularly heavy or painful.

Later on, miscarriage may be signaled by bleeding from the vagina together with contractions of the uterus. Even bleeding alone can be very frightening and upsetting. Not much can be done conventionally to help, but you will be advised to go to bed and rest. This may help and at least you will feel that you are doing everything you can to save the baby, although there is no evidence to show that bed rest alters the miscarriage rate, and healthy babies are born to mothers who have not been able to rest while bleeding. Miscarriage is more likely when there is bright red bleeding, uterine contractions, and an open cervix. As a short-term measure, alcohol will inhibit or slow down contractions.

At least 50 percent of all miscarriages are due to nature discarding a fetus with abnormalities. The process of fertilization and subsequent pregnancy is enormously complex and inevitably does not always take place perfectly. However, you are more likely to be unhappy that your baby has not survived than to be consoled by the thought that it might have had an abnormality.

If you know that you are pregnant and the bleeding and contractions continue until spontaneous abortion (as miscarriage is technically known) takes place, you may find that you know when the fetus has been passed. However, it is not always evident even when a miscarriage is complete, because sometimes the fetus is reabsorbed. If the miscarriage occurs early in the pregnancy, the fetus can look like a lump of hard, whitish or grayish tissue, distinguishable from dark red clots of menstrual blood (the tissue has a different texture and will not be absorbed into soft toilet paper). A later miscarriage produces a fetus that is recognizably human. If the baby has died some time ago, it may be smaller than expected for the dates and less well developed. Ultrasound has a place here, because it can be used to tell whether or not the fetus is still alive despite the bleeding.

If you do miscarry, it can be helpful to keep everything that comes away (known as the products of conception), so that a doctor can see if any tissue has been retained. If it has, you might need a dilatation and curettage to completely clear the uterus.

You will generally be admitted to the hospital when you miscarry, although women who have miscarried before sometimes find they are happier if they stay at home and manage everything themselves.

Nowadays you may find that you are given the option to go home and miscarry naturally after being told that the baby has died. This may lessen the risk of infection and give you welcome privacy and a greater feeling of control at a time when you feel your body is out of your control. If you choose this course, ask for guidelines on what to expect and when you might need medical help.

If you have miscarried and find that the subsequent blood loss smells putrid, or have abdominal pain, flulike symptoms, or a fever, get medical help straightaway because you may have developed an infection (septicemia) that could put your chances of future childbearing at risk.

If you are Rh negative and your partner is not, it is important to have an injection of Rhogam following a birth, a miscarriage, or even a threatened miscarriage, in order to prevent developing antibodies to Rh positive blood, which might harm subsequent children.

If you have experienced bleeding during pregnancy, it is best to avoid intercourse for at least two weeks after the bleeding has stopped. If you miscarry more than once, it may be best to avoid sex until the sixteenth week of pregnancy.

There are some good alternative treatments for a threatened miscarriage, although it is important to note that such treatments will not retain a damaged fetus.

Acupuncture

If you are bleeding in early pregnancy, an acupuncturist will treat you twice within a twenty-four- to thirty-six-hour period, which should stop the bleeding. He will then correct the deficiency and see you weekly for about a month. You may be given moxa (a slow-burning herb used to apply heat to acupuncture points) to use at home, and you may also be advised about diet and rest.

Bach Flower Remedies

Take a few drops of Rescue Remedy (see page 10) in a glass of water. This is particularly good for dealing with shock at the first sight of bleeding.

Cranial Osteopathy

A cranial osteopath can help prevent a miscarriage by working viscerally, through the abdominal wall, to calm down the contractions of the uterus.

Herbal Medicine

Any of the following herbal remedies may help:

- False unicorn root (*Chamaelireum luteum*)—half an ounce (15 g) to a pint (600 ml) of water, boiled and simmered gently for fifteen minutes. Drink copious amounts. Alternatively try two to three drops of the tincture, three times a day.
- Wild yam root—take two to four ounces (50 to 120 ml) of infusion every half hour. The tincture is said to be less successful and may cause vomiting. Take ten drops every half hour.
- Lobelia tincture—no more than fifteen drops in a small glass of water every fifteen minutes as needed.

Homeopathy

Treatment for an incomplete miscarriage is Secale and Pyrogen. For septicemia with feverishness and evil-smelling discharge, take Pyrogen. There are several remedies for those who do not recover completely afterward; consult a homeopath. See pages 51–53.

Massage

A gentle massage can help to bring down the heart rate and open veins and arteries so they can work to capacity. Make a massage oil from fifteen drops of clary sage in two ounces (50 ml) of olive oil to help relieve the pain and anxiety, and use it with some of the massage techniques on pages 106–108.

Nutritional Supplements

- Vitamin E (up to 2,000 I.U.s per day)
- Zinc (25 mg, or 15 mg elemental zinc)

- Manganese chloride or amino-chelate (10 to 20 mg)
- Essential fatty acids (1 to 4 g Efamol per day)

Miscarriage, Recurrent

Miscarrying repeatedly is very distressing indeed. Even one miscarriage causes you to doubt your body and feel anxiety about subsequent pregnancies, but when it keeps on happening, your feelings of hopelessness and despair can be quite overwhelming. There are orthodox treatments, such as hormone injections, running a stitch around the cervix if weakness is causing it to open prematurely, and other newer and successful techniques.

Alternatives are well worth considering for this problem. Conventionally, you are only deemed to have a problem after a third or subsequent miscarriage, but you may well want to try to find a solution before you reach this point.

Acupuncture

Nearly all the conditions for recurrent miscarriage are treatable by acupuncture.

Liz was in her late thirties and had had two miscarriages at ten and twelve weeks. She visited an acupuncturist who diagnosed too little blood and a tendency to flush everything out. She was treated and given advice about her diet. Her recurrent headaches ceased and she had no more attacks of herpes. Within two months she was pregnant and with further treatment carried the baby to term. When the baby was overdue, her labor was started by acupuncture. She felt in the peak of health throughout pregnancy and gave birth to a healthy boy.

Aromatherapy

Avoid using lavender, clary sage, or fennel oil. (Although lavender oil is mild enough to use during pregnancy, it should not be used on the skin if there is a threat of miscarriage.)

Herbal Medicine

Take one or two cups of black haw root *(Viburnum prunifolium)* tea daily from the start of the pregnancy. Another recommendation is to take three drops of the tincture of false unicorn root *(Chamaelirium luteum)* four or five times a day from a month before conception until the fourteenth week of pregnancy.

Homeopathy

If there is a tendency to abort at the second or third month, it is well worth consulting a homeopath.

Nutritional Supplements

Take the supplements recommended for a first miscarriage for at least a month prior to conception, and follow the preconception advice in Chapter 3.

MORNING SICKNESS

Morning sickness—which can, in fact, occur at any time of the day and sometimes night—is absolutely miserable. It can vary from intermittent mild nausea to permanent nausea and constant vomiting. It may even consist of sudden vomiting without nausea. In general it is limited to a period starting any time from days or weeks after conception until the end of the first trimester or so, although some unfortunate women have it throughout pregnancy. Even knowing that it is likely to end is not much help if you feel as if you are dying and pregnancy has just been confirmed. It is more common in those expecting their first child, a girl, or more than one baby. Although it makes you feel appalling, be assured that retching and a lack of appetite will not damage the baby. Research has shown that the fetus will take the vital nutrients it needs from its mother at any expense. The baby will not suffer even though you are.

There are a lot of suggestions about what might help this unpleasant condition. If one remedy does not work, try another. Start by

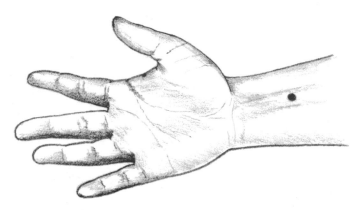

Acupuncture point to stop morning sickness. Apply pressure to a point on your wrist, three fingers down from the wrist crease in between the two tendons.

looking at ways in which changing your routine might improve the problem.

- Keep a glass of apple juice beside your bed, so that you can sip some in the night and have a drink first thing in the morning.
- If possible have herbal tea and dry crackers brought to you in bed, and get up gradually.
- Eat small, bland, easily prepared meals frequently.
- Rest as much as possible, in bed whenever there is the chance.
- Exercise regularly—a brisk walk can help alleviate feelings of nausea.

Acupunture

Acupuncture works well on the special points for stopping sickness, or you could buy a band marketed for seasickness which applies pressure to one of the points. Alternatively, you can make your own by strapping a pebble tightly onto the inside of your wrist, three fingers down from your wrist crease and in between your two tendons. One study showed a 60 percent improvement in morning sickness in women who used acupressure like this.[2]

Aromatherapy

Lavender, chamomile, rose, and ginger essential oils may make you feel better. Lavender and ginger are antiemetic and antispasmodic and can be used as a massage oil or in a warm bath or in a compress placed over the abdomen.

Herbal Medicine

Ginger has a good reputation as a remedy for nausea of any kind. It can be taken in any form—as tablets, a few drops of essence or tincture, crystallized, as ginger beer or an infusion made with fresh shredded root or ordinary powdered ginger.

Other herbs that may help if taken as infusions are chamomile, peppermint, hops, lemon balm, meadowsweet, black horehound *(Ballota nigra)*, gentian, and raspberry leaf. Peppermint can also be taken as one drop of essential oil on a sugar cube.

Homeopathy

Think about your symptoms and how you are feeling generally, then see how they match those given below. The remedy that describes your symptoms most accurately is the one to try.

Ipecac—constant nausea and/or vomiting that is not relieved by vomiting; clean tongue; may be irritable and probably suffer from loss of appetite; feel worse lying down.

Sepia—feelings of nausea are worse in the mornings; can't bear the smell or sight of food or cooking; no loss of appetite, and indeed symptoms may be relieved by food; may experience an empty feeling in stomach and possibly feel depressed or indifferent.

Ant. tart.—spasmodic vomiting of undigested food and mucus immediately after eating; exhaustion or collapse; may be worse in the evening and better from sitting upright.

Nux vomica—spasmodic vomiting after breakfast; bitter taste in the stomach; stomach feels as though it contains a heavy weight; may be constipated and be irritable.

Arg. nit.—nausea and vomiting with flatulence; experience a craving for sweet things; want fresh air; worse from heat and may be anxious or panicky.

Nutritional Supplements

Specific supplements may help, if you are not already taking them.

- Vitamin B_6 (10 to 100 mg per day)
- Magnesium (200 to 400 mg per day)
- Zinc sulfate (25 mg per day, or 15 mg elemental zinc)—seems particularly helpful
- Brewer's yeast (two heaped teaspoonfuls may be mixed with milk and mashed banana)
- Vitamin K injections

Vitamin B_6, taken as a 25-mg tablet every eight hours, has been shown to have a significant effect in reducing or stopping severe nausea and vomiting. The effect was noticeable within three days.[3]

Osteopathy

Consider this if bending over a sink or the toilet causes pain in your back. Problems in the dorsal spine can affect the vagus nerve leading to the stomach, which when irritated can cause vomiting.

Reflexology

Reflexologists report a good success rate in relieving the nausea and vomiting of pregnancy.

NASAL CONGESTION

Some women seem to have a blocked nose throughout pregnancy due to relaxed blood vessels in the nose caused by the increase in progesterone. Unfortunately, there is not much that can be done about this because it is part of the general facial swelling, although putting a few drops of eucalyptus or peppermint oil onto a handkerchief may help. Rosemary oil in an essential oil diffuser can clear the air and make breathing easier.

Women are often concerned that a cold will prevent them from using breathing techniques in labor. Quite often the nose clears during labor, though the cold returns after the birth.

Nose Bleeds

These are also common in pregnancy because of the increased amount of blood in your system. They can be stopped by putting a cold compress containing a drop of lavender or cypress oil over the bridge of your nose.

Posterior Babies

This is when the baby's back is against your back so that its limbs are toward the front. One sign may be that you have a saucer-shaped dip around your navel. It is a position that can make labor longer and more painful and gives rise to a lot of backache. If the baby does not turn during the course of labor—most do—it can mean that forceps are needed.

To try and shift the baby, spend a lot of time on all fours; the weight of the baby's head should swing the rest of it round. Use this position in labor too. Crawling may help.

Premature Labor

Going into labor at any time before about thirty-seven weeks can be very frightening. You may realize that labor is starting if you are getting regular contractions, which may feel like aches or constrictions in the abdomen, aches in the back, or stronger versions of the Braxton–Hicks contractions that you may already be used to. Premature labor can also start with bleeding or rupture of the membranes. If you are not due for a long time yet, you might think that your stomach is upset or that you are suffering from indigestion.

However, if you think you might be in labor, call your midwife, doctor, or hospital for instructions. You might ask if they recommend a stiff drink—alcohol can inhibit contractions. If you are certain that you are in labor, call an ambulance because premature labor can be quite rapid and premature babies do need hospital facilities. If the baby is going to be very premature, i.e., less than thirty weeks, it is best to get to a hospital with neonatal intensive care facilities. It can be easier to move a very premature baby before birth, rather than afterward. If you are trying to prevent an imminent birth while traveling to a hospital, adopt the knee-chest position: Kneel with your bottom high in the air and your head on your crossed arms.

In some women painful, regular contractions occur for varying lengths of time throughout pregnancy. If this happens to you, wash your hands thoroughly and check that your cervix is not dilating, then rest with a hot water bottle to ease the pain. If membranes have broken, do not check internally in order to prevent infection. Seek help immediately if your cervix is dilating.

When traveling long distances by car during late pregnancy, remember to stop and walk around every couple of hours or so. Sitting still for long periods seems to encourage stronger Braxton–Hicks contractions in order to pump blood around the uterus. If you are susceptible, this could trigger premature labor. One British obstetrician reports unusually high numbers of premature births in women who have driven to Devon from the North of England without a break.

Herbal Medicine

Try taking motherwort tincture—as much as is needed to stop contractions. You can also try small amounts of a decoction of false unicorn root—half an ounce (15 g) to a pint (600 ml) of water, simmered for fifteen minutes. Other remedies include taking a decoction of cramp bark *(Viburnum opulus)* or black haw *(Viburnum prunifolium)*. Wild yam *(Dioscorea villosa, paniculata,* and *mexicana* as well as related species) is useful for uterine pain (not premature labor) in pregnancy. Simmer one to two teaspoons wild yam root in one cup of water for ten to fifteen minutes. Drink this three times a day or take tincture (2–4 ml) twice a day.

Homeopathy

Treat the cause; see the remedies for miscarriage, on pages 76–79. If the membranes have ruptured, take Arnica. When the pains begin, take Sabina.

Membranes that rupture prematurely, often at the time of a growth spurt at thirty-two weeks, can heal if you rest.

PRESSURE OF THE BABY'S HEAD ON YOUR PELVIS

The baby's head can press on nerves in your pelvis, causing discomfort. This usually passes as the baby shifts position, but occasionally it becomes stuck in an awkward position and becomes a real problem. The homeopathic remedy for this is Bellis perennis 6x. Acupuncture and osteopathy may also help or you can try sitting back on your heels and tipping your pelvis back and forth. This exercise may move the baby and ease pressure on the bladder.

SACROILIAC JOINT PAIN

This can be an agonizing pain caused by the loosening of the ligaments, allowing the two sides of the sacroiliac joint to move and grate together. It is felt low down on the back just under the dimples above the buttocks. It causes pain on turning over in bed and climbing stairs and can be quite crippling. Osteopathy is the best treatment, but reflexology can help too.

Sciatic Nerve Pain

This is a pain that radiates down your thigh and can cause great discomfort. It can be improved with treatment by an osteopath or chiropractor or by massage with Nelson–Bach's Rhus tox. cream. Some women have found that using a TNS machine can help (see page 108).

Aromatherapy

Treat as an inflammatory condition and rub in massage oil with lavender. You could also apply a compress of sweet marjoram or German or Roman chamomile.

Skin Discoloration

Women sometimes develop a discoloration of the skin on the face in pregnancy, traditionally known as a butterfly mask. It can appear as a brownish stain that covers the nose and parts of the cheeks. Generally the discoloration fades slowly after the birth. There does not seem to be much that can be done about it, although it has been suggested that supplements of PABA, para-aminobenzoic acid, may help (up to 500 mg per day). It is found naturally in wheatgerm, whole grains, liver, mushrooms, fresh fruit, and vegetables.

It is usual for a brown line to appear on the abdomen from the top of the pubic hair line to the navel.

Stretch Marks

Once stretch marks appear as purplish lines over the breasts or abdomen, they are permanent, although they will fade to a silvery white. They can be prevented by rubbing on a mixture made by combining one ounce of wheatgerm oil with thirteen ounces of sweet almond oil and adding to it:

twenty-five drops lavender
five drops neroli
five drops frankincense
five drops lemongrass

Massage daily into thighs, buttocks, breasts, abdomen, and upper arms after a bath.

Varicose Veins

Varicose veins can appear for the first time in pregnancy, and often get worse in subsequent pregnancies. They may appear in your legs or vulva and cause considerable discomfort by aching and itching. They can be apparent as bulging, bluish veins under the skin or may ache without being especially visible. The right leg is often the worst affected.

You can help yourself by putting on support tights *before* you get out of bed in the morning—this gives the veins support before gravity increases the pressure of blood within them. Walking is helpful, too, because it aids the return of blood to your heart. Squatting is not recommended. Instead, lie on your back on a rug or cushion with your legs up the wall. In fact, try to lie with your legs higher than your head whenever possible.

Vulval varicose veins may be more comfortable if you wear a sanitary pad in well-fitting underpants. Soak it in cypress oil and water for additional relief. If there is no improvement, the veins may need to be cauterized.

Aromatherapy

Massaging the veins gently with diluted cypress oil will help shrink them. Also try adding a few drops of lemon and cypress oils to your bath.

Homeopathy

For aching legs that feel bruised and strained, take Arnica. If your legs are weary and feel as if you can't walk, take Bellis perennis. If you have varicose veins as well and your legs feel bruised and sore and congested, take Hamamelis.

Nutritional Supplements

Take extra vitamin E (300 to 600 I.U.s per day) together with one to six garlic perles.

YEAST INFECTION *(CANDIDA ALBICANS)*

A vaginal yeast infection causes a white curdy discharge and intense itching that can make your skin very sore. It is caused by a yeast that is present in everyone but on occasion proliferates and becomes out of control.

It is more common during pregnancy because the fungus thrives on the sweeter, moister condition of the vagina in pregnancy. It is generally treated with antifungal pessaries that treat the symptoms but may not prevent a recurrence.

If you get frequent infections, you should consider whether you might be one of the many people that suffer from systemic candida. This is a condition in which the immune system has become weakened and candida is able to gain control of the body. This can occur following the use of antibiotics, the Pill, or steroids. Even eating meat that has been treated by antibiotics can trigger the condition. Symptoms can include recurrent vaginal yeast infections or cystitis, endometriosis, athlete's foot, allergies, abdominal bloating, diarrhea or constipation, premenstual syndrome, depression, lethargy, poor memory, muscle aches, tingling, numbness or burning, aches and swellings in the joints, menstrual cramps, spots before the eyes, and loss of libido. You may be a sufferer if you are adversely affected by the smell of perfumes, tobacco smoke, or chemicals, or if you crave sweet foods, bread, or alcohol.

Candida is treatable, but it may require several months on a diet which avoids the yeasty and sugary foods that "feed" the fungus. Ideally this should be before you become pregnant, but it can be done while you are pregnant provided you are very careful to balance your diet.

The process can be speeded up by taking supplements that encourage the growth of healthy intestinal flora and create an environment that is hostile to candida. Oral Nystatin can be prescribed by your doctor, which will speed the process, but this is best taken before you become pregnant.

The foods that should be avoided are bread, cakes, cookies, anything breaded, mushrooms, soy sauce, sour cream, black tea, all cheeses, citric acid, dried fruit, alcohol, malted products, vinegars, anything containing sugar, smoked or preserved meats or fish, and nuts that have not been freshly cracked. Fresh fruit should be avoided for the first three weeks because of its high sugar content. Do not take any nutritional supplements that are not stated to be yeast-free.

It is quite probable that you may feel worse as the candida starts to die off, but this feeling will pass after several days. You can help yourself still further by eating live, natural yogurt, taking capsules of lactobacillus daily (available in a nondairy form for those allergic to milk), and perhaps taking some acidophilus or Probion. Take two or more garlic perles daily as well as a zinc supplement (25 mg, or 15 mg elemental zinc, daily).

Candida overgrowth is more common in women who are deficient in zinc, iron, or both. Detailed advice on remedies are available in the excellent book *Nutritional Medicine*, by Dr. Stephen Davies and Dr. Alan Stewart, published by Pan.

A Scandinavian study showed that applying yogurt to the vagina cured infections in women during the first three months of pregnancy, when they were reluctant to use anything systemic that could have affected the baby.[4]

Aromatherapy

This remedy is adapted from Maggie Tisserand's recipe for a vaginal douche for yeast infection from her book *Aromatherapy for Women. While a douche is absolutely contraindicated during pregnancy,* it can help to take a sitz bath in two pints (1.2 liters) of warm water to which two drops of rose, four drops of lavender, and two drops of bergamot have been added. Stir well.

Another remedy is to sit alternately in bowls of hot and cold water to which a teaspoonful of the antifungal thyme and tea tree oils have been added.

Herbal Medicine

First insert two Probion tablets into the vagina. (Replace tablets twice a day until improvement.) Eat live natural (unsweetened) yogurt daily. You can dab yogurt directly on the afflicted parts or, if not pregnant, douche with a mixture of one quarter cup yogurt to one quart of water. Or apply undiluted yogurt using an applicator or tampon. Take at least three garlic perles twice a day and eat as much raw garlic as you can manage. Drink raspberry leaf tea instead of black tea and completely cut out sugar in any form, including alcohol. A poultice made from slippery elm bark powder and water, backed with muslin, and applied to the vulva can be soothing.

Garlic suppositories can be very effective (in lieu of Probion). Peel a clove of garlic, wrap it in thin gauze, and insert it into the vagina. Repeat for several days, changing the suppository every few hours. Babies can be born with candida (see pages 194–195) and thus may inherit a weakened immune system. Also try eating sprouted wheat, either fresh or as tablets, daily.

Homeopathy

Nat. phos. 6x tissue salt may help or try Candida 30.

8

The Birth

You will have many questions in late pregnancy. How and when will labor start? What will it be like? Will I be able to cope or will I let myself down? It is impossible to make accurate predictions about anything to do with childbirth. You should remember this when someone tells you that you will have the baby by next week or lunchtime, or that it will be a difficult or easy birth, or that the baby will be huge or tiny. You can only go by the way that you feel. It is better to avoid asking for estimates about any of these things because people are notoriously wrong, and you may be basing your course of action on a guess.

However, here are some guidelines that may enable you to find the answers to your questions about your own labor.

INDICATIONS THAT LABOR IS STARTING

Labor starts when the level of progesterone in the body falls and the level of estrogen rises. This can result in any of the following symptoms, but it is important to remember that labor can often seem to begin only for all the signs to die away for another few days or even weeks. You will feel less frustrated if you play down early symptoms so that there is a minimum of fuss when it turns out not to be labor at all.

Weight Loss

A decrease in the amount of amniotic fluid can mean that you lose about two to three pounds (1 to 1.5 kg) in the last few days before labor. You may find that you can feel your baby more distinctly through your abdominal wall.

The Baby Moves Less

Toward the end of the pregnancy the baby has much less room to move, and you will feel fewer kicks than you did, say, at thirty-two weeks. In the last few days the baby may slow down still more. If it kicks less than ten times in twelve hours, speak to your midwife, doctor, or hospital. They will want to monitor the baby, probably on a cardiotocograph or belt monitor.

Nesting Instinct

This is the famous urge to rush around preparing your nest for the imminent arrival of the baby—for some reason it often seems to manifest itself in a desire to clean the oven! If you are affected by this instinct, make sure that you conserve your energy so that you are not completely exhausted by the time contractions start.

Diarrhea or Stomach Upset

Many women report having to make numerous trips to the bathroom at the start of their labors. It seems to be nature's way of clearing the bowel so that a full rectum does not impede the baby's passage down the birth canal.

Feeling Different

Sometimes women wake feeling different, maybe better or worse than usual. Women have described having flulike symptoms, feeling irritable, extra uncomfortable, or even brilliantly well.

Bloody Show

A mucus plug fills the cervix during pregnancy and acts as a barrier between the vagina and the baby and the membranes. As your cervix changes shape at the beginning of labor, the plug is loosened and comes away; you may find the "show" in your underpants or on the toilet paper. It can appear like a lump of sticky, clear jelly that may be streaked with blood making it appear pink, although some women find that theirs is quite loose and runny. Occasionally there is a small amount of blood with it, caused by the membranes becoming detached from the wall of the uterus. If it is bright red and enough to soak a pad, call your midwife or hospital.

Rupture of the Membranes

This is one of the things that can cause anxiety. Most women find that their membranes—the tough bag that contains the baby and the surrounding amniotic fluid—rupture at home, but many worry that it will happen when they are out. This isn't as embarrassing as it might seem, and no one will think that you have wet yourself. In fact, most people will be unlikely to notice.

When the membranes rupture, it may be with an audible pop or ping and a feeling that something has "broken." It will be followed by a gush or a trickle depending on the size of the rupture and the position of the baby within your pelvis. The fluid has a distinctive smell, which helps to distinguish it from urine, and you may notice an increase in the flow at the time of Braxton–Hicks or true contractions. The membranes often break while you're in bed, which is why women are often advised to sleep on waterproof sheeting, although this can make you unpleasantly sticky.

Labor usually starts within some hours of the membranes going. If you know the baby's head is engaged in the pelvis, you need only put on a pad to soak up the fluid and carry on quietly as normal.

Contractions can start almost immediately or may take as long as several days to get going. Conventionally, obstetricians like babies to be delivered within twenty-four hours of spontaneous rupture of membranes, and will want to induce you if labor is not well under way by then (see page 111). This is because there can be an increased risk of infection to you or the baby from bacteria traveling up the vagina. Some will allow you to wait longer, providing you take antibiotics. Some midwives take a more relaxed view and will wait as long as six days before considering induction.

If you do not want to be induced, try taking eight garlic perles and vitamin C (1 g) several times a day to combat infection, and be scrupulous about hygiene. This means showering instead of bathing, being careful to wipe from front to back, and not introducing anything into the vagina (no vaginal examinations or sex). Try any of the methods of self-induction that do not involve contact with the vagina (see pages 113–115). If your temperature is raised, you may well have an infection that must be treated.

There are two situations in which you need to take immediate action following ruptured membranes. One is if you know the baby's head is high (i.e., not well into the pelvis) or if you are not sure if it is engaged. The other is if the amniotic fluid that drains away is stained with meconium—the greenish black contents of the baby's bowel. It might be any shade from green through brown to black. Fresh meconium, which might have been passed as a result of the baby being currently in distress, is green. It causes concern when it is thick because there is a risk that the baby may inhale it.

The risk with membranes rupturing while the head is still high is that there is a very slight chance that the umbilical cord might precede the baby's head into the birth canal. As contractions push the head downward, the cord can become pinched between the baby's head and the pelvis, cutting off the baby's blood supply. This only happens in one out of four hundred deliveries, and it is much more likely to happen when the membranes are ruptured artificially.

In both these cases you should immediately call your midwife, doctor, or hospital. If you know the head to be high, try and lie flat until you have been examined. If the cord is definitely protruding, call an ambulance straight away and lie face down with your knees on the ground and your bottom high in the air. Do not touch the cord except to push it carefully back into your vagina with clean hands.

Change in Cervix

Cervical changes provide the most convincing evidence that labor has started. If you are accustomed to feeling your cervix regularly, you will be in a good position to notice the way it changes toward the end of pregnancy. A "rip" cervix—one ready for labor—feels soft and malleable, more like your lips to touch than your nose. It will have become softer, shorter, and thinner and you may be able to insert a finger easily.

If you think you are in labor, you can make sure by feeling your cervix. *You must wash your hands thoroughly first* (see page 32). If your cervix is high or you can't reach it, you are unlikely to be in labor because the cervix descends and becomes easier to reach as it dilates. At this point, if it is accessible, it will feel as if the edges are frayed. It may feel wobbly, and you may be able to get two fingers inside.

When you are definitely in labor, the baby's head moves down, and you will feel the cervix lower in your vagina. There will be nothing left of the canal of the cervix; it will have been taken up into the body of the uterus so that all that remains is the tissue stretched over the head, with the os or opening gradually getting wider. At this stage it may feel like something slimy over a grapefruit. It may be stretched taut so that you are unable to get your fingers inside it, or you may feel the plasticlike membranes with the amniotic fluid behind them. The hole left by the dilating cervix is completely round, and once it is fully dilated (10 cm), there is no rim of cervix left at all.

The chief advantage in doing your own vaginal examination is to make sure you are in established labor (usually 3 to 4 cm dilated) before taking your next step. There can be an interval of quite some hours between the start of contractions and reaching this stage, especially if it is your first baby.

Contractions

Many, but not all, women are aware of contractions of the uterus from about twenty weeks of pregnancy onward. In fact, the uterus is contracting at intervals throughout our lives. You may experience these contractions, known as Braxton–Hicks, as occasions during late pregnancy in which the uterus seems to swell and become hard and tight. The contraction lasts for about a minute and can make walking difficult.

Braxton–Hicks contractions tend to occur more often if you are exercising or if you have been sitting still for a long time.

Toward the end of pregnancy, these contractions can occur more frequently, last longer, and start to become uncomfortable. At this stage they may be starting to prepare you for labor by effacing your cervix. Quite often you can get a spell of harder contractions with shorter intervals between them, which then fade away just when you are convinced it is labor. If this happens during the night, it can be helpful to have a warm bath or a cup of chamomile tea or perhaps a couple of acetaminophen or a mild alcoholic drink *(do not mix the two)*. This will not stop labor but will let you get a night's sleep if it is not labor.

Labor contractions become more frequent, last longer, and are stronger. They may start by feeling like period pains or give you backache, or radiate down your thighs. The classic pattern is for them to start at half-hourly intervals, then gradually to come at intervals of twenty minutes, fifteen and so on, until they are lasting up to two minutes with as little as a one minute interval between them. Of course not everyone fits this pattern; some may have contractions at five minute intervals until the end, or they may last the same length of time or the contractions may come at irregular intervals.

When to Go to the Hospital

If you are having your baby in a hospital, you will want to know when to go. This will obviously depend on circumstances such as how far away you live and whether you are likely to get caught up in rush-hour traffic, whether you have other children to be cared for, and so on. However, it may be time to go if:

- You are in labor before thirty-six weeks.
- You are bleeding, even a heavy show.
- You are in labor and your previous births were very quick (see Chapter 9, "Precipitate Labor"), although this is a good indication for home birth.

- Your membranes have ruptured and the baby's head is high, or the amniotic fluid is colored (see page 94).
- You are more than 5 cm dilated.
- You feel you cannot cope or are very frightened.
- Contractions are every five minutes or more often and last longer than a minute, providing that you also feel that you need to go now.

It is obviously very difficult to gauge how strong the contractions are if this is your first labor, and the risk is that you will go in too early, thus increasing the chances for intervention. It is best to hang on until you feel you absolutely cannot manage at home any longer. Try not to err on the safe side, and if you find that you are only slightly dilated when you get to the hospital, go home again.

LABOR

Labor itself consists of uterine contractions that initially alter the shape of the uterus from a bag with a neck hanging down into the vagina to one unit, forming the birth canal. The contractions then change from those that dilate the cervix, to being expulsive in nature with the top of the uterus exerting pressure downward, forcing the baby out through the vagina. This simple explanation belies what can be a process that may take many hours, be extremely painful, and totally exhausting. It tends to go much more smoothly if you are happy in your surroundings, feel supported, and are confident that you are in good hands. It can be more difficult if you are frightened, miserable, unhappy, and do not feel at home in your situation or with those who are with you.

The First Stage

The first stage of labor can take any time from days to minutes, although it is wise to allow twenty-four hours. In the early phase it can be exhilarating—you are finally about to experience the event you have been awaiting for so long. At first you can get on with things normally, and you are able to talk through contractions. It is best to play down the drama at this point and save your "breathing" until later. If it is nighttime, find something to do that will take your mind off labor since everything appears more intense at night. Concentrating on something else can be very useful at this stage.

As the contractions get stronger, you will find that you have to devote more attention to them and that you become less interested in what is going on around you. It may help to breathe through the contractions, using a simple technique of breathing in through the nose and out through the mouth *slowly*, concentrating on the outward breath, and deliberately relaxing your body. It also helps to keep mobile and remain in an upright position, perhaps rotating your hips like a belly dancer. By now you may feel that labor is a serious business, and you may be surprised by how painful the contractions are becoming, although you will probably feel fine in between.

Toward the end of the first stage of labor (when the cervix is between 7 and 10 cm dilated) some women experience a phase known as transition. This is a combination of a physical and mental state where your legs might tremble, you may get cramps in them or your bottom; you may vomit or feel that you need to push before you are fully dilated. Mentally it can be a confusing time when you may feel that you can't cope any more, that the whole thing is a bad idea, and that you will give it up for the time being and resume later. You can be very irritable, swearing at everyone and wanting to go home even if you are already there. It can be a low point, when you feel as if you have used up all your energy and you are in despair.

The Second Stage

The transition can last from minutes to a couple of hours and some women never experience it. It ends when the cervix is fully dilated, which may coincide with feeling the urge to push. This sensation, which is initially felt at the height of a contraction, can be so overwhelming that you can do nothing but go with it. If you do not feel it, your body may be in a resting phase that can last up to half an hour. It is a mistake to start pushing before your body is ready.

Pushing should come naturally if you have had a drug-free labor and are in an upright position. However, this does not mean that it will not be hard work—it can require every ounce of your effort. It can help to make several short efforts with each contraction, deliberately relaxing your pelvic floor and pushing down with your diaphragm. It helps to visualize the baby coming down and round the curve of the birth canal. It can be a long process when the baby seems to move five steps forward and four back.

A squatting position, or supported squat, can be a good position for delivery, because there is no pressure on your coccyx to impede progress and gravity assists the downward movement. The all-fours position can help to control a rapid delivery and is a good position during labor if the baby is posterior (has its back against your back with its limbs facing out), because it can assist the baby to turn and present more favorably.

Some people find the second stage of labor, from full dilation to the birth, very painful, and others welcome the opportunity to do something positive after a long period of allowing the body to do most of the work. Quite a few women describe the moment of crowning, when the baby's head comes through the stretched perineum, as being like splitting, burning, or bursting. Your midwife may tell you to pant rather than to push at this point; if you can, you have a better chance of not tearing. You can guard your perineum with your hands—this may also help if you have difficulty knowing exactly in which direction to push.

In the majority of births the baby's head will emerge facing toward your anus and then rotate so that it faces your thigh. The baby's upper shoulder is helped to slide underneath the pubic arch, followed by the lower shoulder, and then the rest of the body slithers out.

When you first see your baby, she may look blue purple until she takes her first breath, when she rapidly turns pink. The baby can be quite slippery and messy and may still be covered in vernix, the white waterproof cream that protects the skin while in the amniotic fluid. The baby may look waterlogged or streaked with blood and mucus and have a thick blue and white cord coming from the navel. The genitals of either sex can be astonishingly prominent. The baby's head may have been molded during birth so that it looks most unnatural and is swollen around the eyes. Breastfeeding is most likely to succeed if the baby is put to your breast immediately.

The Third Stage

You may overlook the final stage of labor in the excitement of meeting your baby at last. The emotions felt at this time and stimulation of the baby's nursing results in the production of oxytocin from the pituitary gland into the bloodstream. This causes the uterus to contract and become smaller and the placenta to separate from the uterine wall. Further contractions should ensure that the placenta is delivered soon after the baby. It resembles a large piece of liver.

PAIN RELIEF IN LABOR—THE OPTIONS

Nearly every woman finds labor very painful and feels at some point that she would like something to relieve the pain. Among the pharmacological methods available for pain relief are inhalation gases, such as nitrous oxide and ether, narcotics, such as Demerol or Meptid, and epidural anesthesia. All have some disadvantages and most are only available in the hospital.

All drugs taken during a woman's pregnancy and labor cross the placenta and affect the baby to greater or lesser degrees, depending on the drug and the amount taken. Each woman needs to inform herself thoroughly about the potential risks of drugs commonly used for pain relief in order to make an informed decision based on her own personal situation, and each woman deserves to have her choices respected by her doctor or midwife. Be sure to ask your birth attendant for more information about which methods of pain relief are likely to be offered as you labor, and read about the subject on your own (see the suggested reading list on pages 199–203, especially *The Birth Machine* by Marsden Wagner).

There are alternative ways of relieving the pain of childbirth. Few can remove the pain completely, but they are free from side effects to you and your baby. All of them are more effective if you have plenty of support and encouragement. One study concluded that good support is equal to a full dose of Demerol in its ability to reduce the appreciation of pain. Some simple measures that might help include using a hot water bottle on your back or front, and massage. Try taking a calcium supplement (about 200 mg daily) at the start of labor in order to provide a boost of calcium to compensate for the large amounts required by the contracting muscles. If preferred, effervescent calcium can be taken in water (1 g every three hours).

Acupressure

You may find some of the following techniques useful for relieving the pain of labor or speeding it up if it is protracted.

- Place your thumbs over the acupressure point indicated, using the balls of your thumb rather than the tips. Place your weight over them.
- You will find that the points are more sensitive than the surrounding areas; some have slight indentations underneath them.
- As the mother breathes out, build up pressure steadily and evenly over the acupressure point. Maintain the pressure while she holds her breath for three to seven seconds and then release the pressure as she breathes out. Then move on to the next point.
- You can also use your elbow gently—this can be useful for large areas such as the buttocks or shoulder muscles.
- If you use your fingers, put your index finger on top of your middle finger for more depth. This is useful if you find that your thumbs are getting tired.

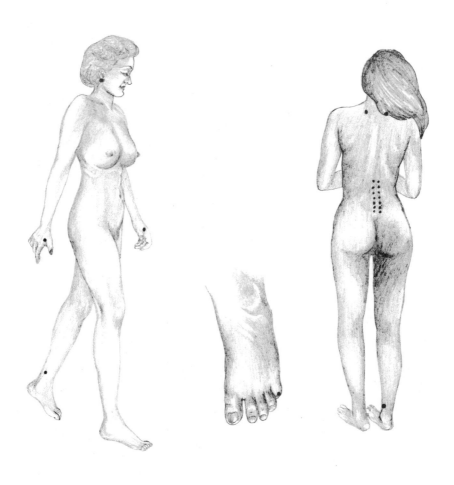

Acupressure points to relieve pain during labor.

Points to help relieve pain and speed labor (see figure on page 102):

1. On the web of skin between the index finger and the thumb (colon 4). This should only be used for labor; if it is used before it could cause miscarriage.
2. In the groove behind the shin bone, three of the mother's thumb widths above the ankle prominence (spleen 6).
3. Bladder points either side of the spine, one and a half inches from the groove of the spine, from waist-level to her coccyx.
4. The inside of the ankle between the ankle prominence and Achilles tendon (kidney 3). This is good for both postpartum hemorrhage and retained placenta.
5. Points between C7 and the achromium process. Massage all the way along from the point indicated out to the tip of the shoulder—this can be very useful if labor is slow.
6. Massage the point at the outer edge of the nail of the little toe at the base of the nail. This may be easier if done with a matchstick.

Caroline's water broke on Tuesday evening when she was almost forty weeks pregnant, and she had no contractions. She wanted to avoid induction and asked the hospital doctors not to intervene. She stayed in the hospital at their request, but by Thursday afternoon she had still not had any contractions and her doctors were insisting on induction of labor the following morning. Late that afternoon, she tried stimulating as many of the acupressure points that she could reach and continued to do so until she went to bed. Nothing seemed to change but she woke at 1:00 A.M. in strong labor and in less than two hours she gave birth to a healthy girl, who weighed eight pounds, eleven ounces.

Acupuncture

If you can have an acupuncturist with you in labor, he or she can relieve the pain and speed up the labor if necessary. They can also stop any nausea. It takes about ten minutes to work and does not remove pain completely, but reduces it to a bearable level. Transcutaneous electronic nerve stimulation has a similar effect.

Aromatherapy

Try adding a couple of drops of clove oil to a warm bath at the start of labor to ease the pain.

You can make a massage oil to relieve pain and tension in labor by combining:

two ounces sweet almond oil
ten drops lavender
six drops clary sage
four drops geranium
two drops jasmine
three drops rose

This can be massaged onto any part of the body and smells wonderful. The smell can raise the spirits of all who are present.

A compress made by dipping a cloth into a bowl of hot water to which a few drops of clary sage have been added can relieve the intensity of contractions. Wring out the cloth and hold it over your pubic bone.

Herbal Medicine

Coriander is recommended by Juliette de Bairacli Levy in her book *The Illustrated Herbal Handbook.* She suggests taking three or four sprays of leaves eaten raw as a salad herb; taking half a teaspoon of the seeds mixed with honey and eaten raw; or making a tea from the seeds. Raspberry leaf tea can be drunk freely throughout labor, or it can be taken as previously prepared ice cubes. Poppyhead tea can also help with pain relief—take six fresh or dried poppyheads in one-half pint (300 ml) of water. Susun Weed, herbalist and author of *Wise Woman Herbal for the Childbearing Year*, recommends three drops of skullcap and twenty-five drops of St. Johnswort tinctures taken every hour if needed.

Homeopathy

In preparation for labor, you may want to buy a selection of remedies from a homeopathic pharmacy. Although homeopaths often differ in their recommendations for remedies, you and your birth partner may find this guide useful.

Caulophyllum 200x—Take when contractions are ineffective or the cervix too rigid to open. Use it when contractions are sharp and spasmodic, the mother is exhausted, weak, and sensitive to cold.

Sarah was expecting her second baby; she was four days overdue and had been given a date for induction a week later. She was anxious for labor to begin and at midnight her membranes ruptured. She went to the hospital and stayed in but only had twelve contractions all night. The doctors were going to induce labor if it did not begin within twenty-four hours.

At 10:30 A.M. she started taking Caulophyllum 30x every half hour, and she also stimulated her nipples for about fifteen minutes. Within an hour contractions were coming every five minutes. She continued taking the Caulophyllum and at about 3:15 had treatment from a reflexologist. Sarah noticed a distinct increase in the strength of contractions following the reflexology, and labor was well under way At 5:45 she had a girl, who weighed seven pounds, seven ounces.

Pulsatilla 200x—This should be taken when contractions begin and then stop and are ineffective. The mother is weepy and thirstless, needs attention and air, and may be begging for help. It can also be useful for turning a malpositioned baby.

Kali. carb. 30x—Take this for pains in the back, buttocks or thighs when the mother wants her back pressed hard. She may be sweaty, weak, anxious or irritable, or have a headache—this remedy may need to be repeated frequently.

Chamomilla 200x—This should be taken when the mother is angry and irritable; she can't bear the contractions or to be examined. She may kick, swear, or strike someone. Contractions can seem to be forcing the baby up, rather than down, and the mother may have pains in her thighs.

Cimicifuga 200x—Mother is frightened (see also Aconite) and despairing, feels out of control. She is restless and talkative. Contractions may be better if she lies on her left side.

Massage

Massage is a wonderful technique for relieving pain and tension because it relaxes muscles and induces a feeling of well-being. It is useful during pregnancy to ease aches and pains, improve the circulation, aid digestion, and stimulate the lymphatic system.

In labor massage is probably the most helpful way that a partner can help to ease pain and reduce the feelings of isolation that women sometimes get. Massaging someone can relax the donor as well as the recipient, and fathers often appreciate having something constructive and effective to do. It can be helpful to practice the techniques before labor starts, but it is not essential.

If you are giving the massage, you should:

- Use cornstarch-based body powder or oil (see page 104 for massage oil for labor recipe) to reduce friction.
- Breathe in a relaxed way, breathing from the abdomen. The laboring woman will pick up your breathing rhythm.
- Rest your hands on her for thirty seconds before starting.
- Massage toward the heart—upward from the legs, downward from the shoulders.
- Always keep one hand on her body.
- Try to establish a rhythm so that is feels like a continuously flowing stroke.
- Vary the pressure—lighter over bones, firmer over large areas of muscle.
- Ask her to let you know if it is not helping—you need to be very responsive, sensations can alter by the minute in labor.
- When the mother is on all fours, support her head in one hand

while you massage her back with the other. Make sure you are well-braced to support the weight of her head. If she relaxes into this position, you will find her head heavy.

- Women often twist one foot against another in labor—it can help just to hold each one firmly.
- Stroke up her forehead into her hairline gently, with one hand following the other in a rhythmic sequence.
- Press your thumbs firmly into the center of the buttocks to relieve backache.
- Support one foot with one hand and stroke the sole firmly with the heel of your other hand.
- Apply deep pressure with your thumbs in a line down the center of the sole to the heel.

Some massage techniques that are helpful in labor:

- Using both hands, stroke gently but firmly from the shoulders down to the fingertips.
- Place your hands on her shoulders and massage her neck and shoulders with your thumbs.
- Massage down her back, starting at the shoulders down to the base of her spine—one hand should follow the other in a continuous motion.
- Keeping your fingers on her hips, use your thumbs to rub hard into the bony area around the sacrum.
- Pushing the heel of your hand hard against the base of the spine and rubbing it in a circular motion so that the skin moves over the bone and there is no friction between the skin and the spine—this is very good for backache. (It can still be done with TNS electrodes in place but there should be less need for it.)
- Firmly massage the inner or outer thighs upward, concentrating on the inner thigh.
- Very lightly massage with fingertips under the belly, starting well up one side, going underneath, and coming up on the other side. This technique is either welcome or irritating.

- When you end the massage, take your hands off slowly making it obvious by a change in rhythm that you are about to stop.

Massage needs to be done in a smooth, rhythmic sequence. However, bear in mind that women sometimes cannot bear to be touched while they are in labor or find that some types of massage that were previously enjoyed are unhelpful, so you need to be sensitive to her changing needs.

Transcutaneous Electronic Nerve Stimulation

The machine used for this method of pain relief is available in some hospitals and can also be rented. It is a small battery-operated device that delivers a minute charge of electricity to the nerves that supply the uterus at the point where they enter the spine. It works by stimulating endorphins—the body's natural opiates—and by helping to prevent the message of pain from reaching the brain. Four electrodes covered in conductive gel are taped to your back and connected to the TNS machine by means of a lead. A push-button handset allows you to alter the mode of operation between the on-off mode, which gives an intermittent pulse and is used between contractions, and a continuous mode used during contractions. A dial allows you to increase the impulse.

It is best used from the onset of labor and takes about twenty minutes to work. The sensation is a bit like "pins and needles." Most women find it helpful and some need no other pain relief.

The disadvantage is that it cannot be used with a bath or shower, and it may interfere with a fetal scalp monitor. If you intend to use a hospital machine, you either have to go in early in order to use it or risk putting it on later than would otherwise be ideal.

Postpartum Hemorrhage

Ipecac 200x—first choice. Arnica 200x—second choice.

After the Birth

Aconite 30x—Give this to the baby if shocked, blue, or fails to urinate. Give three to four doses in the first twenty-four hours of life. (This remedy is also very useful for mothers or fathers who feel very fearful during the labor.)

Calendula tincture—Take this tincture diluted in water (one part tincture to twenty parts water) or chamomile tea for episiotomy or tears. The water must be first boiled and then cooled.

Bellis perennis 30x—If the uterus feels sore, squeezed, or congested, take one tablet a day for three days.

Arnica 200x—Take twice daily after birth to help soft tissues heal.

You should take each contraction as it comes and know that you are coping well if you manage with that one. It is not a good idea to dwell on how you cannot stand another few hours of labor because childbirth is entirely unpredictable, and even experienced midwives can be wrong in their predictions of how long your labor will last. Basing your decisions on estimates can mean that you choose forms of pain relief that you would prefer not to use. You do, however, need to keep an open mind because labor can be far more painful than you anticipate.

9

When Labor Is Not Straightforward

INDUCTION

Labor is sometimes induced for sound medical reasons, such as if the mother's blood pressure is high and continuing to rise, or the baby is hardly moving, or there is proven growth retardation. However, induction is often pressed because the consultant has a policy of inducing everyone who is a certain number of days overdue; this can even be on the due date in certain cases or it might be as long as two or three weeks.[1] Some consultants do not induce without a medical indication, and surveys are beginning to show that mothers and babies fare better without this intervention. Labor goes most smoothly when it is spontaneous.

There will always be a reason given for your induction, but keep in mind that you can resist the offer if you want. There is no consensus on the risks of prolonged labor and the stage at which you are considered dangerously overdue will depend on where you are having the baby. You may like to have the baby's heartbeat monitored on a cardiotocograph, a belt monitor that will trace its heart readings and your contractions if any. Regular monitoring for periods of half an hour will show how well the baby is withstanding the rigors of life in utero.

Medical induction can consist of the following measures:

- Sweep of membranes—This is when a midwife or doctor inserts a finger into your cervix and sweeps it around the top, detaching the lower membranes. This often initiates labor, but it can only be done if your cervix is already ripe.[2]
- Prostin pessary—This is a pessary containing prostaglandins which is given in the hospital to ripen the cervix with the aim of starting labor. It is often given the night before a full induction and can send you into spontaneous labor.
- Artificial rupture of the membranes—Membranes are ruptured by means of an amnihook which looks like a plastic crochet hook and is inserted through the cervix to snag the membranes and release the amniotic fluid. This often starts labor and is also used to accelerate a labor that has started spontaneously. The disadvantages, apart from the fact that it is done in a hospital, are that it can be very painful if the cervix is not ripe; it might thrust you suddenly into very strong labor; and most consultants are committed to deliver you within twenty-four hours, if necessary by cesarean section, due to the resulting risk of infection.
- Pitocin drip—This is synthetic oxytocin administered intravenously into the arm. This may be used if other methods have failed or it may be put up at the same time as the membranes are ruptured. It usually starts contractions, the strength of which can be controlled by altering the amount of Pitocin. The disadvantages are that artificially stimulated contractions can be a lot harder to cope with than natural ones and lead you to other interventions. You may need more pain relief than you otherwise would. If you have an epidural, you are more likely to need forceps. You will be asked to accept continuous monitor-

ing because there is a risk of overstimulation of the uterus. Pitocin creates a greater risk of your baby becoming jaundiced or requiring special care, and if it fails, your baby will be delivered by cesarean section.

Alternatives to Induction

These alternative methods for triggering an overdue labor are not foolproof but have a certain amount of success and are well worth trying if you think that you are going to have to agree to a medical induction.

- Sex—Semen contains prostaglandin and can work in the same way as the Prostin pessary, although the prostaglandin is less concentrated in semen. Frequent sex, followed by lying on your back with a pillow under your bottom for at least half an hour can therefore sometimes start labor.
- Nipple stimulation—Stimulating your nipples for fifteen minutes or more at a time stimulates the release of oxytocin and thus labor.
- Curry—This is a purgative working on the same principle as castor oil, but rather more palatable. Have as hot a curry as you can stand.
- Castor oil—Take a third of a tumbler mixed well with liver salts or orange juice. Unfortunately, it is unpleasant to take and is followed by violent diarrhea. However, it can start labor if you are on the brink, and it clears the bowel so that you will not need a suppository, but if it works you may start labor feeling rather weak.
- Sweep of membranes (see page 112)—You can try stretching your cervix manually yourself.
- Homeopathic remedy—Take Caulophyllum 30x every half hour until contractions start. If this works, keep taking the tablets until labor is well-established, otherwise labor may be long, drawn out, and sluggish.

  One midwife reports good results in encouraging labor by the use of one tablet Caulophyllum 200x dissolved in a glass of cold water. The mother drinks two-thirds of the water and then tops it off repeatedly, so that it becomes increasingly dilute and thus more powerful in homeopathic terms.

One of her clients had had painful, irregular contractions for ten nights. Although they were sufficiently painful to warrant using a TNS machine, she was not yet in established labor, although she was understandably becoming demoralized. Her cervix was 3 cm dilated and still thick.

The midwives suggested taking Pulsatilla 10M (a very powerful potency only available from homeopathic pharmacies), which in their experience either postpones or stimulates labor. In this case it took the woman out of labor so she was able to eat, drink, and have a good sleep. They left the Caulophyllum remedy, and she called them back about four hours later. When they arrived she was huddled in a chair feeling tearful—this suggested that labor might have progressed and she was in fact 6 cm dilated. The baby was born two hours later.

- Acupuncture—Treatment from an acupuncturist does work although it can take several treatments over three to four days. An acupuncturist may put in a retaining pin that stays in the skin so that you can apply pressure on the point yourself.
- Cranial osteopathy—A cranial osteopath can get labor started by working via your pituitary gland, although it takes a couple of days to take effect.
- Herbal remedies—Goldenseal is an oxytocic herb. Try taking twenty drops of the tincture every hour until contractions are regular. It is extremely bitter, so have something sweet ready to suck after taking it. Labor tincture is a recipe from *The Wise Woman Herbal for the Childbearing Year* by Susun Weed. It might be wise to make up this herbal remedy at least six weeks before you are due if you think you are at risk of induction. You will need:

  one-half ounce (15 g) dried black cohosh root
  one-half ounce (15 g) dried blue cohosh root

> one-quarter ounce (10 g) dried ginger
> one-quarter ounce (10 g) dried beth root
> eleven ounces (325 ml) vodka

Put the dried herbs in a large, opaque jar and add the vodka. Label the jar clearly and cap it. Allow the mixture to steep for at least six weeks. When you want to decant it, put it into a juice extractor or pour into a muslin cloth and squeeze out as much liquid as you can. Store in a brown glass container in a cool dark place. Alternatively, you could buy the tinctures from an herbalist and combine them. When the tincture is required, take ten drops under the tongue every hour until contractions are regular. Castor oil rubbed into the abdomen and covered with a warm towel may also help trigger labor if the cervix is ripe. (See Sarah's story on page 105.)

EPISIOTOMY

An episiotomy is a cut made into your perineum (the skin between the vagina and the anus) in order to enlarge the outlet for the baby. It is one of the aspects of childbirth that is most dreaded and disliked. It is done when the baby's head is stretching the perineum, by infusing the area with local anesthetic and then cutting it with very sharp scissors. The cut is made from the vagina outward and backward, slanting away from the rectum. It may be done without an anesthetic in an emergency because the perineum is numbed naturally by the stretching.

Some of the reasons for performing an episiotomy include fetal distress, a "rigid" perineum that is holding the baby in, or a forceps delivery for whatever reason. In addition, some doctors will tell you that an episiotomy is better if it looks as if you might tear or that "all first-time mothers in this hospital have episiotomies and all subsequent mothers who have had episiotomy previously must have a repeat." Many doctors are not used to doing deliveries without them.

Clearly some reasons have more validity than others, and you are dependent to some extent on the skill of your attendants. Some midwives take a particular pride in delivering so that a cut or tear is avoided. A tear may be preferred to a cut if damage is inevitable because it will follow the natural stress line instead of cutting through the muscle and because it heals better and more comfortably. The edges, being irregular, knit together like a jigsaw. Moreover, you have the slight satisfaction of knowing that if you tear a bit, at least you have avoided a routine episiotomy. Make sure your attendants know if you would prefer to tear; you are not always asked before an episiotomy is done. Some midwives feel that tears heal best with few or no stitches. The bruising and blood loss will be minimized, and there will be fewer problems with infection and healing if you take Arnica 200x immediately before and after delivery.

Obviously, prevention is better than cure, and there are a number of ways of avoiding the problem. The first is the long-term measure of perineal massage (see pages 43–44) and the second is by taking care at the time of birth. This can be done by applying a washcloth wrung out in hot water to the perineum to soften the tissues. Massaging the perineum with oil in the second stage can also help the baby to slide out without trauma. When the baby's head crowns, you need to control your breathing so that you stop pushing and allow the head to slip out. Your midwife may ask you to pant, and it is vital to do this although you may well feel that you are past caring. The more slowly the head emerges, the greater the opportunity for the perineum to stretch and accommodate it. You can help by reaching down to feel your baby's head and helping to guide it out while supporting your perineum (but it is difficult to do both by yourself).

The position that you deliver in can make a difference to your chances of tearing—upright, squatting, or all fours positions are best, all fours probably providing the best opportunity for control. Lying flat or semisitting is more likely to result in damage. There may be a higher incidence of tears among mothers who give birth in water.[3]

If the baby does need help to be born, ask that vacuum extraction be used in preference to forceps. In experienced hands, this means less risk of damage to the baby's head and requires less of an episiotomy or possibly no episiotomy at all.

If you do have stitches, they may not necessarily bother you, but they can cause enormous pain and discomfort, making the postpartum period miserable. At its worst, sitting can be so painful that it is impossible to find a comfortable position in which to feed the baby, and some women are forced to nurse standing up.

The pain does diminish in the end and your perineum heals over, although it can be a deterrent to sex for quite a while. Making love with the pressure off the scar and using KY jelly may help, but if your scar is not comfortable by the time of your postnatal check, make sure that your doctor appreciates the fact. Occasionally, poor stitching needs redoing. Make sure that you get a midwife or experienced doctor to suture you, and beware: medical students first learn to suture on perineums!

Practical tips include applying ice packs or bags of frozen peas to the area, throwing a handful of salt into your bath as an antiseptic, taking the pressure off by sitting on an inflatable rubber ring (available from a drug store), alternately sitting in a basin of hot and cold water, and drying stitches (after washing) with a hair dryer. Ultrasound treatment can increase the inflammatory phase and stimulate the healing process.

Aromatherapy

There is a very valuable remedy that combines lavender and cypress oils in equal quantities. Add six drops of the mixture to water in a sitz bath or large bowl and sit in it as long as needed. You can add more drops if your skin will tolerate it.

Jane had an episiotomy for the birth of her daughter and suffered a third-degree tear and two internal tears. Nothing prescribed by the hospital brought any relief, but trying this remedy in the bath once she was home worked well to relieve pain and assist healing.

Her doctor initially thought that the tears would need to be operated on for further repair and was impressed that they healed spontaneously with the help of the essential oils and calendula tincture.

Herbal Medicine

Bathe the wound with a few drops of calendula tincture in warm water or use the solution in a spray.

You can also make a paste with slippery elm bark and water, olive oil, vitamin E oil, and comfrey powder if you have it. Spread it onto muslin and hold it in place with a pad. Change it every time you use the bathroom. Once the wound has healed, try massaging the scar with vitamin E or comfrey oil.

Homeopathy

Take Arnica 200x; this will need to be followed by Calendula for some days. If the episiotomy was done against your wishes, take Staphysagria. For intense, burning pains take one dose of Causticum 30x twice daily for four days.

Arnica cream (not ointment) around the stitch line will help ease bruising. Calendula or Hypercal cream will also assist healing.

FORCEPS DELIVERY

Forceps are needed to help a baby out in around 5 percent of births, although they may be used far more frequently. They can be needed in cases of fetal distress, maternal exhaustion, and when the baby's head is well down into the pelvis but progress has halted, frequently when an epidural is in use. They are occasionally used for premature babies and breech births, and to deliver babies born by cesarean section.

If forceps are suggested, it is likely to be at a point where you may be at your lowest, having been pushing for some time, and you may feel that you do not care what is done to you. It is, however, worth making a superhuman effort to avoid forceps. This means getting into a squatting position—even if you have had an epidural anesthetic and cannot feel your legs. Ask those around you to support you, and hold on to the end of the bed.

Some hospitals have policies about the length of time that you are allowed in the second stage before they use forceps. This may be as little as an hour for a first baby and a half hour for a second. You should be allowed as long as it takes, provided you and the baby are coping. It helps to wait until the urge to push is overwhelming; remember there may be a resting phase of as much as a half hour between full dilatation and feeling the need to push. Pushing when the baby's head is high or when you do not want to makes forceps more likely.

A forceps delivery is performed by a doctor while you lie flat on your back on the delivery bed. Your legs are placed in stirrups on either side, your perineum is injected with local anesthetic, and an episiotomy is performed. Once the anesthetic takes effect, both blades of the forceps are inserted into your vagina separately. They consist of a hollow metal guard that curves round the baby's head and a shaft which is angled to go around the curve of the birth canal.

Once the blades are in position, they are locked together so that the head cannot be crushed. With each contraction the doctor pulls and you push; sometimes it requires an astonishing amount of effort. Once the head is out, you push your baby's body out yourself. The resulting depression of the temporal bones may mean that the baby is slow to start to breathe.

Delivery by forceps can cause quite severe bruising and a very sore perineum. You will probably want to try the remedies for episiotomy (see pages 117–118) and take Arnica at the time followed by Calendula for several days, together with Bellis perennis for soft tissue injury and Staphysagria for emotions and shock.

Bach Flower Remedies

The baby can be helped with Bach flower remedies—Star of Bethlehem for trauma and Walnut to help it adjust to change. Mix as recommended on page 10 and drop into the mouth.

Cranial Osteopathy

A baby delivered by forceps would benefit from treatment from a cranial osteopath when it is fourteen days old.

Homeopathy

The homeopathic remedies are Arnica, and if after that the baby is fractious and twitchy, it should be given Kali. phos. 6x.

Failure of Labor to Progress or Slow Labor

This occurs when labor begins and you are having regular, painful contractions, but the cervix fails to dilate. It may not dilate at all, or it may get to some stage below full dilatation (10 cm) and then stop. The causes can include not being able to "let go" because you are frightened or the atmosphere is inhibiting, progress being halted by epidural anaesthesia, and occasionally disproportion when your pelvis is not big enough to birth this particular baby.

If you feel inhibited by the atmosphere or by particular birth attendants, you or your partner will have to have the courage to alter the situation. It is not surprising that many labors slow down or stop as soon as couples reach the hospital, because you may feel on alien territory there, uncertain about what is going on and among people you do not know. The same thing can happen when someone you feel is not sympathetic comes to your home when you are in labor. If progress has stopped, ask everyone to leave you alone for at least fifteen minutes—if necessary leave the hospital and go home. This can be just as effective and a lot more pleasant than having a Pitocin drip put up, the orthodox remedy in this case. It might help to have a bath or a glass of wine or beer. Tell yourself "open" and visualize your cervix opening up. Make sure you keep altering your position and that you are being massaged. Nipple rolling or stimulation stimulates oxytocin and can encourage labor too. If you are in a hospital, you may request a different doctor if you are not getting along well with the one on duty. The chances are that if you are not seeing eye to eye, he or she will be glad of a change too.

If an epidural seems to have stopped progress, you will have to allow it to wear off and then not have it renewed, which may be difficult to accept. Demerol is useful in this instance because it can often relax you enough for the cervix to dilate. The usual approach in a hospital is to further stimulate contractions by means of a Pitocin drip, and, if that fails, to deliver the baby by cesarean section.

Acupressure

Apply pressure from your nail or a matchstick to bladder 67, the point beside the nail of your little toe. Also, see page 102.

Aromatherapy

A bath with a few drops of clary sage, being a euphoric, or massage with clary sage oil in the base, will also help labor along. Also, see page 104.

Herbal Medicine

You could try taking one-quarter to one-half teaspoonful of beth root tincture. Or ten to twenty drops of blue and black cohosh roots—these two should be combined and not used singly. If you have the labor tincture ready made (see pages 114–115), take ten drops under the tongue at half-hour intervals.

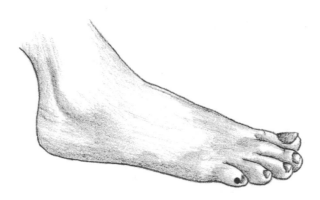

Acupressure point to stimulate contractions. Apply pressure to the point beside your little toenail with a matchstick or your nail.

Homeopathy

If the contractions are changeable, dilation is slow, and you are tearful, take Pulsatilla. If the contractions are relaxed, you are getting "false pains," tiring, or slowing down, take Gelsemium.

Veronica was expecting her second baby. Her previous child had been delivered with forceps after a long labor, and it had been suggested that her pelvis was inadequate. Her water broke at 4:00 P.M., and she went to the hospital at midnight. By 2:00 A.M. labor was established, but at 3:00 contractions stopped. By 4:00 there were still no contractions, and she was threatened with a Pitocin drip. By this time Veronica was anxious but not frightened. The anxiety was treated with Aconite. She was also given Caulophyllum 6x every fifteen minutes. By 4:45 strong contractions were under way, and at 6:30 the baby was born without problems. By 7:30 the placenta had not been delivered (synthetic oxytocin and ergometrine were not given), and the hospital staff were becoming anxious. Caulophyllum 200x was given as a single dose, and the placenta arrived ten minutes later.

Reflexology

Use reflexology to encourage a sluggish labor by holding a strong comb in each hand during a contraction and gripping them tightly so that they press on the midfinger tips and the balls of the hands. It may also help to have someone apply firm pressure to the center of the balls of your feet.

Exhaustion in Labor

Labor can be extremely tiring, which is why it is an advantage to be as fit as possible at the start. It is exhausting to be intermittently in severe pain, and even if you are totally relaxed throughout, your body is still using up large amounts of energy. Long before the end you can feel that you have had enough and would be happy to call it a day. Since this option is unlikely to be open to you, you need to consider the others. The best way to conserve energy is to relax through contractions and, if this proves impossible, to rest completely between them. Relaxation techniques are taught in most prenatal classes.

Exhaustion is frequently exacerbated by a policy of not feeding a woman in labor. This is thought to be safer in the event that you need a general anesthetic, because you are at risk of suffocating if you inhale vomit. However, it is now known that it is more dangerous to inhale the acid that accumulates in the stomach if you are not allowed to eat than to inhale partially digested food. It seems probable that starving laboring women does more harm in leaving them exhausted so that they need more intervention.

In many cases the digestion tends to shut down during labor, and any food you do eat should be light and easily digested. If your system cannot cope with what you have eaten, it will send it back. One remedy is to take fructose—fruit sugar—in drinks or powdered. Fructose is preferable to glucose because it provides a sustained release of energy instead of an initial peak followed by a low. Fructose is available from health food stores.

Demerol can help you get some sleep if you are completely exhausted, although you may find you wake up in the middle of a contraction, unprepared for it and unable to cope. When you are feeling discouraged, you may agree to procedures that beforehand you felt certain you did not want. Obviously, you should be free to change your mind as the situation demands, but it can be useful for a partner to be aware of the possible state of mind that exhaustion brings and to be very sympathetic and encouraging. You can sometimes regret giving in, although it is hard afterward to remember just how little strength you may have felt you had.

Aromatherapy

See labor oil on page 107.

Bach Flower Remedies

Take Rescue Remedy frequently as labor progresses. You might also add Olive and Oak flower remedies.

Herbal Medicine

Herbal remedies include taking tincture of either ginger or wild ginger, either as fifteen to twenty drops in water or as two to five drops under the tongue. Drinking raspberry leaf tea throughout the labor can speed it up. The other herb that might help is pure ginseng; take two to four capsules every four hours.

Homeopathy

For ineffectual contractions that are exhausting and not getting anywhere, take Caulophyllum. For exhausting contractions and labor that is going on too long, take Kali. phos. and Rescue Remedy. These can be taken all the way through if necessary. For doubling up and shivering in the first stage, take Cimicifuga. For transition—unbearable pains, you are irritable or capricious, and feel worse with warmth—take Chamomilla. If the pain is made much worse by the slightest movement or touch, and you want to go home, take Bryonia. In the second stage when the head appears with each contraction, only to disappear again, take Silica. For exhaustion, take Kali. phos.

Stephanie was having her first baby at home. Labor progressed normally for eight hours. Suddenly the pains became intolerable, nothing was right, she wanted rubbing, then she didn't, all positions were uncomfortable—in short she was in transition. She was given Chamomilla 6x with each contraction. An hour later she started to push, was having strong contractions, and was fully dilated. An hour later she was still pushing and not feeling too tired. Another hour passed, and she was still pushing and getting tired in the squatting position; the midwives were starting to think about "doing something." The baby's heart was fine. Arnica 200x was given as a single dose. A half hour later the baby's head appeared with each push, only to disappear again. She took a single dose of Silica 200x and the baby was born fifteen minutes later. The placenta came away forty-five minutes later. Stephanie was very bruised from pushing so long and so took Arnica 200x immediately after the birth and another dose later.

PRECIPITATE LABOR

It can happen that you go into labor very rapidly. This is much more likely to occur if this is not your first baby. There are effective delaying tactics, but the best remedy is for you to feel confident that you can deliver the baby yourself. If labor proceeds that rapidly, nature is working at its best and there is very rarely any problem with either mother or baby.

If you feel that your baby is arriving suddenly (overwhelming desire to push, great sensation of something like a grapefruit in the rectum), call your birth attendant or an ambulance. You can delay the birth by adopting the knee-chest position with your bottom high in the air and your head on your crossed arms on the floor. You can do this on the back seat of a car if you are en route to the hospital. It is important to remember that all that is necessary is to catch the baby and keep him warm until you get help.

If you are delivering your own baby in an emergency:

- Find a towel or blanket to wrap the baby in—it is vital that the baby is kept warm.
- Find a soft spot on which to deliver, and put a towel down if possible.
- When you feel the baby's head coming through your perineum, cup it with your hand.
- Once the head is out, feel for any loops of cord around the neck and bring the cord forward. The baby's head will probably emerge facing your anus and then rotate to face your thigh.
- Wipe the baby's eyes and mouth free of mucus with a clean hanky or your finger.
- Wait for the next contraction, and with it, guide the baby's head down so that its upper shoulder can slide underneath your pubic arch and, once it is free, guide the head upward so the lower shoulder can be freed and its body will follow.
- Wrap the baby up warmly as soon as possible and put him to the breast.

- The placenta will probably emerge within a half hour, especially if you are upright and feeding the baby. If no help has arrived by the time the placenta has been delivered, wrap it separately from the baby and keep the two together. Do not cut or tie the cord.
- If you have not already done so, send for help. Take Rescue Remedy for shock! A baby that has been born very quickly may benefit from taking Arnica for the shock. If the baby shows signs of being fractious in the first weeks of life, consider cranial osteopathy (see page 10–11).

FAILURE OF BABY TO BREATHE

The seconds before the baby breathes can seem an age. If the baby is blue or purple at birth, she will definitely breathe within a minute or so. Occasionally, however, a baby may be white or gray in color and not start to breathe spontaneously. If she is not breathing a minute after birth, she will be given oxygen from a mask. If that does not work, a tube will be put into the lungs to push air directly into them.

If the baby is born unexpectedly at home and fails to breathe, which is most unlikely, there are steps that you can take. First, if possible call medical help. Make sure that you have wiped any mucus out of the baby's mouth with your finger, or suck it out with a straw and tip the baby so that any remaining mucus can drain out of her mouth. Do not cut the cord because the baby needs all the oxygen she can get from the placenta while the cord is pulsing. Stroke the baby's back and tell her why you want her here and flick the soles of her feet with your fingers. You can put a few drops of Rescue Remedy into the baby's mouth and on the pulse points at wrist and temples. Perform mouth-to-mouth resuscitation (see pages 190–191). Don't give up hope—babies can survive undamaged for twelve minutes without oxygen and may start breathing voluntarily.

POSTPARTUM HEMORRHAGE

Heavy bleeding after the baby is born can be terrifying. Even a normal amount, considered to be a pint (500 ml) or less, seems like a lot. If the hemorrhage, which can be either a gush or a persistent trickle, starts shortly after the birth, your midwife or doctor will give you an intravenous injection of ergometrine. This has the effect of contracting your uterus and the site of the bleeding within forty seconds. If you lose a lot of blood, you will require a blood transfusion. Occasionally, a hemorrhage will occur in the two or three weeks following the birth. In this case consult your birth attendant immediately.

Alternative remedies for hemorrhage include chewing a piece of placenta if it has been delivered or pinching your ankle hard at the point between your ankle bones.

Herbal Medicine

Take twenty drops of blue cohosh or labor tincture (see pages 114–115), together with fifty drops of ground ivy tincture. Repeat after two to five minutes as necessary.

Sip half a cup of warm water in which a teaspoonful of cayenne has been dissolved.

Homeopathy

Hemorrhaging is unlikely to occur if you take Arnica and Kali. phos. at birth. If it does occur, see the remedies given for miscarriage with reference to the type of bleeding (see pages 51–53). For bright red bleeding, take Phosphorus. For bleeding accompanied by nausea, take Ipecac. If the bleeding is associated with faintness and dizziness that gets worse with the slightest movement, take Trillium.

CESAREAN SECTION

Between 1970 and 1990 cesarean section rates in the Unites States increased from 5 percent to 25 percent. The national average remains about 25 percent, with some hospitals having a rate of 50 percent or more. It is an operation that, when used appropriately, can save lives and prevent brain damage, but its price can be high in physical, emotional, and financial terms. It should never be regarded as an easy option.

Elective Cesarean Section

There are various reasons why you might be scheduled for an elective cesarean section, that is, one done on a predetermined date. These include: placenta previa, when the placenta blocks the cervix either totally or in part; very high blood pressure that cannot be controlled because induced labor may deprive the baby of oxygen; a previous cesarean section (although this in itself should not be an indication for a repeat cesarean unless the reason for the first one is recurring); a contracted pelvis, when your pelvis is permanently damaged by injury or disease; or a small pelvis, although again this alone is not necessarily a good reason because the dimensions of the pelvis can expand by as much as two inches (5 cm) in labor and most women have the right sized baby for their size; if you want to avoid a cesarean section for this reason, practice squatting, consult a cranial osteopath, and take the remedies for easing delivery given on pages 121–122. If you suffer from herpes, a cesarean delivery will be performed if you have active sores because of the risk of passing the infection on to the baby (see page 70 for remedies for herpes). Another indication for a cesarean section is transverse presentation, when the baby lies horizontally rather than vertically. Some consultants also perform cesarean sections for breech presentations (see pages 53–54).

Emergency Cesarean Section

If a cesarean section becomes necessary during the course of labor, request that the operation be performed under epidural anesthetic. This has two advantages: it is better physically—the baby gets less of the drug and you feel fitter afterward—and it is better emotionally because you see your baby born and have no doubts about it being yours, and you can feed it almost straightaway.

The reasons given for an emergency cesarean section can vary depending on the policy of the doctor and the hospital. Doctors sometimes prefer to deliver by cesarean section if premature labor cannot be stopped, although this is done less frequently as it is now realized that some stress helps the baby to adapt to being born. Other reasons include: placental abruption, when the placenta starts to separate from the wall of the uterus before labor, leading to pain and bleeding; cord prolapse (see page 94), when the cord descends first and is compressed as the baby comes down, cutting off blood supply; and fetal distress, when the baby becomes short of oxygen while still unborn. The distress manifests itself as an alteration in the baby's heart rate, which either becomes very fast—above 160 beats per minute—or too slow, below 100 beats per minute. It is normal for the baby's heartbeat to slow at the same time as contractions, but less healthy for it to slow down once the contraction is over. Distress may also be shown by the baby discharging meconium into the amniotic fluid, although this does not definitely prove that something is wrong.

If your baby is showing signs of distress, you can help by moving on to all fours and breathing oxygen from a mask. If the heartbeat drops suddenly and drastically or gradually deteriorates before you are in the second stage of labor, a cesarean section will be performed to reduce the risks to the baby. Other reasons given for an emergency cesarean section are failure to progress (see pages 120–122); obstructed labor, which occurs when the baby eventually presents abnormally, either by face, brow, or shoulder in a position that cannot be altered or delivered vaginally; failed induction; and failed forceps, when the use of forceps fails to deliver the baby.

After the Operation

Although recovery from a cesarean is relatively rapid, you will, nonetheless, be recovering from a major operation at the same time as starting a demanding career as the mother of a new baby, and it is important for everyone around you to appreciate that fact.

At first the postoperative pain will be controlled by drugs, but within a few days you will find that you can start to manage without them. A TNS electrode either side of the scar can provide drug-free pain relief. You will be encouraged to be up and about within a day or so, although you will still need help to get in and out of bed. It is difficult to stand upright at first because of the alarming but erroneous impression that your stomach is about to fall out through your stitches.

Pillows are invaluable for helping you maintain your position in bed and assisting you to balance the baby in a comfortable position for feeding and cuddling. It can be quite a shock to discover just how little you can do for yourself at first—you may need to hold on to the bed-stead to pull yourself up to a sitting position, and you will certainly need help with turning in bed and feeding the baby.

You will be on a fluid diet at first, progressing quite rapidly to light food. Fruit cordials and soft fruit are very welcome in the early days. The third day after the operation is notorious for being the one in which you will be contorted with enormous amounts of wind. This can be helped by drinking peppermint water, available from the hospital. You can also get a flatus tube so that you make less of a racket. The homeopathic remedy Raphanus 30x is excellent for painful wind re-sulting from a cesarean section.

Although you may feel quite well by the time you leave the hospital, life will be much harder when you get back home so it is essential that you have lots of efficient help.

Acupuncture

Acupuncture is useful to treat a scar that remains painful or does not heal well.

Cranial Osteopathy

Babies delivered by cesarean section can also benefit from cranial oste-opathy, because they need the rhythmic squeeze of contractions to ini-tiate a healthy cranial rhythm.

Homeopathy

Take Arnica followed by Calendula for several days. If the operation was against your wishes take Staphysagria. Spray the wound with Calendula or Hypercal tincture, diluted one part tincture to ten parts water. The baby should have Arnica after birth and Kali. phos. if fractious or twitchy.

10

After Birth

How will you feel immediately after your baby is born? You may feel either elated or exhausted, depending on the circumstances. What you are unlikely to be able to do is sleep, no matter how tired you are. After an initial feeding your baby is likely to fall asleep, leaving you more awake than you have ever been, pondering over and over again recent events. This period of wakefulness seems to be essential for you to be able to make sense of the monumental happenings and life changes that have taken place.

At home this can be a family time, and you will be able to eat and drink exactly what you want. In a hospital, on the other hand, food will be limited to what is available, and you may well be ravenous. However, try and ensure you have some time together as a family, although this will depend on the availability of space in the birthing rooms. Eventually, though, your companions will have to leave the hospital, and you and the baby will be left alone.

Sooner or later you will become aware of the way your body is feeling. Although it is a topic that is not much discussed and something that you do not anticipate when you are still concentrating on how labor will go, the reality of the early postpartum period can be quite a shock. For months, you and the baby have been one large, perhaps uncomfortable, but self-contained unit and then quite suddenly you are separate. You and the baby are likely to feel the difference—you seem to be leaking from every orifice, you will be sweating a lot, starting to leak milk, urinating copiously, and, surprisingly after nine or so blood-free months, bleeding heavily.

The baby too is quite a different proposition. Whether you find your baby adorable or you are still coming to terms with his or her existence—and you may well not fall instantly in love with your infant—he or she will soon need attention too. Babies are often sleepy for the first day or two, but after that they may need feeding every two hours or so, day and night, and even while sleepy they need changing every few hours.

If you have stitches or are very bruised, you may find yourself wishing that you were still pregnant, a thought that would have been incomprehensible only a day or two before. You may feel catapulted into motherhood before you are ready. You feel that you need time to recover yourself before taking on the twenty-four-hour-a-day responsibility for a vulnerable baby, but unless you are very fortunate in your help this rarely happens. Even in the hospital where you do have some expert assistance, the awareness of your baby's dependence on you can prevent you from relaxing and recuperating. Some cultures look after new mothers far better than is common in the West, with mother and baby being cared for by other women and protected from work and worry for four to six weeks. A fascinating account of postpartum rituals in other countries can be read in Alison Parra Bastien's article "Postpartum Rituals: Honoring the Mother" in *Midwifery Today* and Sheila Kitzinger's *Women as Mothers*.

Unless you are prepared for it, you can be appalled to find that the reality after all the months of waiting can be an anticlimax, and that you may be one of the many mothers who go through a period of mourning for their vanished pregnancy and the baby that they imagined theirs was.

BOWELS

Constipation can figure even more prominently when you are newly delivered than during pregnancy—especially if you have had an episiotomy—mainly because there is the anxiety about what will happen to your stitches or your tender perineum when you do manage to open your bowels. The hospital with its routines, none-too private lavatories, and often low standard of hygiene is not the ideal place to resolve the issue either. Many women find it is much better once they get home.

If you have had stitches, do not expect to have a bowel movement before at least the third day. When you think you can brave it, put a clean pad over your stitches to hold them in place. The stitches always do stand the strain, but it is hard to believe it at the time. Other ways of helping are to squat on the toilet seat, to lubricate the rectum with a little baby cream, and to practice your relaxation and breathing techniques at the time. It may help to lean to one side, taking pressure off the stitch line. If the prospect is really terrifying, take painkillers beforehand (be sure to discuss this with your midwife or doctor ahead of time if you are breastfeeding).

Eating food with considerably more fiber than the average hospital diet will help too, but the problem most often is not that you feel no urge but that you dare not obey it. Try the alternative remedies given for constipation in pregnancy (see pages 56–58) to see if they help the problem. Be careful not to take any purgatives such as senna, though, as they can be passed through the breast milk and give the baby diarrhea. Your midwife can supply suppositories or an enema if things get really bad.

Osteopathy can help if the problem becomes long-term which can happen, particularly after a forceps delivery.

PAINFUL COCCYX

The coccyx (tailbone) is displaced backward when the baby passes through the birth canal. If it feels painful afterward or even before the birth, take the homeopathic remedy Hypericum. If the problem lasts longer than a few days and makes sitting painful, you can get help from an osteopath.

REDUCING THE RISK OF INFECTION

Infection is a real risk in hospitals and a not surprising one if you consider that you have a raw wound in your uterus where the placenta used to be. The opportunity for cross-infection is considerable when there is no disinfection of shared lavatories, bidets, and baths between uses.

To reduce the risk of infection have your baby at home or request a private hospital room and leave the hospital as soon as possible after the birth. If this is not possible, be scrupulous about changing your sanitary pad frequently and wiping yourself from front to back after emptying your bowels. Try to keep your stitches dry, but do not share a hair dryer, and keep any contact with the toilet seat to the minimum. Lavender oil is an antiseptic; try adding a drop or two to the bath water. Use disinfectant on the toilet seat, the squeeze bottle, and the bath before using them.

EXCESSIVE BLEEDING

Bleeding can be quite profuse in the early days and gradually tails off as the days go by. The lochia, as it is called, is bright red initially and may contain clots, before slowly turning brownish pink and eventually yellow. It can take as long as six weeks to stop altogether. When you become more active, you may notice that the flow increases and becomes redder. If you get a real gush at any time, contact your midwife (see recommendations for postpartum hemorrhage on page 127). You can control excessive lochia by applying pressure to a point just in front of the webbing between the big toe and the one next to it, on the upper side of the right foot, or consult an acupuncturist.

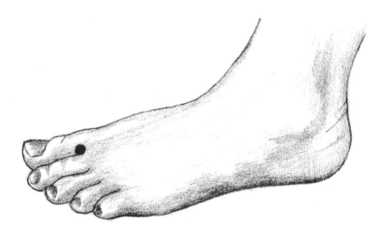

Acupressure point to stop excessive bleeding (lochia). Apply pressure to a point just in from the webbing between the big toe and its neighbor on the upper side of the right foot.

RETAINED TISSUE

Excessive bleeding can be a sign of retained tissue. After birth your placenta and membranes will be examined closely to make sure that no part of them has been left behind. Small pieces of tissue may emerge with the lochia ordinarily, but tissue that is retained for any length of time can cause a problem. It may be responsible for continued bright red bleeding and can give rise to infection, signaled by an evil-smelling discharge and a rise in temperature. Treatment conventionally is by dilation and curettage, a gentle scraping out of the contents of the uterus under general anesthetic. An equally effective but less invasive approach is treatment from an acupuncturist. Arnica taken regularly helps to reduce the amount of blood loss too.

Seek help straight away if you start to feel flulike, have a rise in temperature, or if your lochia starts to smell offensive. A course of antibiotics will probably be needed.

Retained Placenta

Left to itself the placenta should become detached from the wall of the uterus within half an hour of the birth. Sometimes you may need to give a push or two to help it on its way. However, it is standard practice to inject a combination of synthetic oxytocin and ergometrine into the thigh as the baby's shoulder is born, which stimulates the uterus to contract within seven minutes of administration. This reduces the likelihood of postpartum hemorrhage, but increases the possibility of the placenta becoming trapped inside the uterus. If this does happen, the placenta is usually removed manually under general, or occasionally epidural, anesthetic. However, the effect of the drug wears off after two hours, so that waiting is an alternative to operative removal. Patience may also be needed if you decline the injection because placentas sometimes take a while to become detached. If there is no excessive bleeding, there should be no need to do anything else. The cord can be cut once it has stopped pulsating. However, waiting can get tedious and there are ways to speed things up.

Sometimes tension holds the placenta in and relaxing can let it go. Breastfeeding stimulates the uterus to contract and expel the placenta. It also helps to remain upright if at all possible. Drink raspberry leaf tea, squat, and apply pressure to the acupressure point between and below the ankle bone and Achilles tendon on the inside of the right foot. Having a warm bath with your baby can help, as can blowing hard into a bottle.

Acupuncture

Treatment by acupuncture can often be effective as shown in the following case of a home birth:

We didn't want any complications so after what seemed like a long time of sitting on the bedpan, blowing into a bottle, and putting the baby to the breast and the placenta still wouldn't deliver, I had acupuncture on the side of my foot and within minutes it came away.

Aromatherapy

Massage with jasmine oil aids placental separation.

Cranial Osteopathy

A cranial osteopath was called to attend a woman who had given birth but whose placenta had not materialized. He worked on her head and said that it felt as though her sacrum had been pushed up under her ribs. As he held her head, he felt the sacrum suddenly fall back into position and the placenta came away immediately afterward.

Herbal Medicine

Try ground ivy tincture, one-half to one teaspoonful (2.5 to 5 ml) under the tongue. Otherwise try thirty to fifty drops of angelica root—this can be combined with the labor tincture (see pages 114–115). An alternative remedy is one tablespoon of chopped lemon balm leaves eaten raw. Or a large handful of feverfew leaves simmered in two cups of water for three minutes and steeped for three hours.

Homeopathy

Try Caulophyllum, and if it does not work try Pulsatilla, but be patient—it might still take an hour for the placenta to appear.

AFTERPAINS

The uterus continues to contract and shrink in the first week or two after the birth. These contractions are not usually painful following the birth of a first baby but do grow increasingly painful after each subsequent birth. They often coincide with breastfeeding and can be easily as intense as the contractions of labor.

Herbal Medicine

Try taking five to twenty drops of motherwort tincture before feeding the baby or ten to thirty drops catnip tincture, or forty drops of cramp bark tincture, three times a day.

Homeopathy

Arnica taken as a matter of course after the birth may prevent the problem arising. Try Mag. phos. if afterpains do occur.

POSTNATAL DEPRESSION

Some depression is normal after having a baby. However well you may have prepared, you are bound to find the reality of having a baby in your life quite a shock. It demands a huge adjustment in terms of your personal freedom and in the way that you and others see yourself.

However, there is a point at which the normal feelings of inadequacy, tiredness, anxiety, and fearfulness about the baby become postnatal depression. This is an illness that is exclusive to women who have given birth. It may start immediately after the birth or take hold in the following weeks. It varies in severity, being easily recognized at its worst and perhaps missed in its lesser forms. It affects at least on in ten new mothers.

You may be able to diagnose the condition in yourself if you feel that there is no point in getting up, that you are interested in nothing and experience no emotions, or feel unreal, strange, or sad. You may find you have lost your sense of perspective and are very tearful or hysterical and feel overwhelmingly tired or panicky. You could dread going out, feel terrified or suicidal, or worry that you are going mad. You may be waking early, unable to sleep or eat and take to obsessional or compulsive behavior or feel very bored or angry. You may be depressed if you cannot manage to take the baby out of the house or cope with his or her most basic needs. You may feel like you don't love the baby.

If you or your family think that postnatal depression is affecting you, it is important to seek help. One of the characteristics of the disease is, however, a refusal to admit that there is a problem, either because the state seems normal and warranted by the circumstances or because you fear the consequences and stigma of admitting to mental illness and would prefer to recover by yourself. Time does cure it eventually, but in the meantime you are likely to be unable to enjoy the pleasurable side of having a baby.

Orthodox treatment often takes the form of antidepressants, which can be effective but may have a time lag of two weeks before taking effect. Some doctors believe the cause is hormonal and prescribe synthetic hormones to correct the imbalance. Orthodox options may not be acceptable for the breastfeeding mother who does not feel comfortable taking drugs or hormones that will be passed to her child.

Postnatal depression is such a horrible condition that it is often best to consult a practitioner as soon as you can face it. Your partner may need to over-rule your objections if, as is likely, you are in no position to help yourself.

You can get effective treatment by trying one of the alternative therapies. This approach can prove satisfactory even when orthodox treatment has failed.

Acupuncture

Traditional Chinese medicine promotes ten days of bed rest following the birth as essential for the prevention of postnatal depression. If you are depressed, though, you can be treated very successfully by acupuncture.

Bach Flower Remedies

Try a combination of Walnut, Star of Bethlehem, Mimulus (for fear), and Rock Rose (for panic).

Cranial Osteopathy

Cranial osteopaths believe that the illness is caused by the downward displacement of the uterus following birth and a resultant tug on the pituitary gland via the dura. Cranial osteopathy should be effective in helping the problem within two weeks.

Herbal Medicine

You could make your own brew for the treatment of depression according to Susun Weed's recipe in *The Wise Woman Herbal for the Childbearing Year*. This uses:

one-half ounce (15 g) dried, shredded licorice root
one ounce (25 g) dried, crumbled raspberry leaves
one ounce (25 g) dried, finely cut rosemary leaves
one ounce (25 g) dried, cut skullcap

Use two teaspoonfuls of this mixture per cup of boiling water. Take two or more cups daily for as long as is needed.

Homeopathy

Postnatal depression rarely occurs after homeopathic births, but the remedies are as follows:

Simple blues, due to tiredness and excitement—Kali phos.
More severe blues, with indifference, irritability, and lack of maternal feelings, even rejection—Sepia.
Very despondent, changeable, weepy, worse in stuffy rooms, wants fresh air, better with sympathy—Pulsatilla.
Sad, irritable, cries on her own, worse with consolation—Nat. mur.
Listless, sad, and exhausted due to loss of fluids (i.e., hemorrhage or shock)—Phosphoric acid.
Depression and exhaustion due to anemia after hemorrhage—China.

Nutritional Supplements

Postnatal depression may be prevented by eating the placenta. One woman, who had suffered badly after a previous birth, ate hers and found not only that she felt much better and had no recurrence of her symptoms, but that she actually looked a lot better, with supple skin and silky hair whereas previously her skin had become very dry and her hair had fallen out.

She did have a problem overcoming her natural revulsion and initially cooked pieces. She subsequently regretted this when she found that swallowing it raw was no less palatable and likely to be more effective since steroids can be destroyed by heat. She kept the placenta in the refrigerator and cut off small squares, put them at the back of her mouth, and swallowed them. She found it worked instantly as a natural antidepressant. (As nothing has been killed in order to produce it, this option is available to vegetarians too—in theory.)

You could try taking vitamin B$_6$ and evening primrose oil (1 to 4 g per day). Elemental zinc (15 mg) is said to have very impressive results in improving postnatal depression.

11

Breastfeeding

There are two important things to remember about breastfeeding: the first is that correct positioning is vital, and the second is that you can do it if you really want to.

PREPARATION

Your breasts need little preparation for breastfeeding unless, unusually, one or both of your nipples turn inward. In this case you can make a suction device by cutting off the end of a hypodermic syringe and applying suction over the nipple to draw it out before feeding. Shells, worn during pregnancy to help draw out nipples, are now thought not to be of much use.[1] However, breastfeeding is an area in which advisors can be particularly dogmatic, and you should feel free to do what you find helpful rather than what is currently held to be correct.

You should receive help with breastfeeding from your midwife or birth attendant either in the hospital or at home. If you are not getting the help you require, you can get support or advice from breastfeeding counselors in La Leche League. You do not need to belong to this organization to ask for help.

It can be a good idea to rub your nipples with a towel after a bath to make them slightly less sensitive because they can become sore when they suddenly receive a lot of unaccustomed attention after delivery. You may notice quite early in the pregnancy that your nipples exude a yellow fluid. This is colostrum, the substance rich in protein and antibodies that the baby feeds on until the milk comes in. You do not need to express it, but experimenting with your nipple and the areola, the brown area around the nipple, can give you an idea of what the baby's gums will need to stimulate in order to nurse effectively.

Buy several good maternity bras. It can be a relief to start wearing them as early as the fifth month of pregnancy because they are designed to give your breasts extra support.

STARTING TO FEED

It is easiest to put the baby to the breast as soon as he is born, but it is possible that neither of you may feel like it then. Your position is not so important for this first feed, but it is important for the baby to latch on correctly to get a proper feed and to reduce the chances of you developing nipple problems. Bring the baby to the breast by putting your other hand behind its head. Persuade him to open his mouth by stroking his chin with your nipple, and then when it is open, put the whole of the areola, *especially* the lower side, into his mouth. The idea is that the baby feeds from the breast, not the nipple, which should be well back into the baby's mouth. The baby's sucking exerts a powerful vacuum, and if this is misplaced it can damage the nipple, making feeding excruciatingly painful. If the baby has latched on properly, you will be able to see the muscles beside his ears waggle as he feeds. The baby should be allowed to feed for as long as he wants from the breast, but you can detach him when necessary by inserting a finger into his mouth. The milk flow can be stopped by depressing the nipple.

Milk production is initiated by a change in hormones—as the high level of estrogen and progesterone fall following the birth, the level of prolactin rises. Prolactin is responsible for the formation of the milk, which comes in at some time between the second and fifth day. This can happen quite suddenly within a few hours, and you may find that your breasts alter overnight from being soft and comfortable to becoming rock-hard, hot, and tender. They may also be enormously swollen. This engorgement only lasts for a day or two, although it can be very uncomfortable and can cause problems if the baby finds it difficult to latch on. It is at this time that the baby begins to feel hunger and may start crying for food as often as every two hours. This can be quite a taxing stage in your new relationship, and it is important that you rest and do not try to do anything other than get to know each other.

A baby can be beautifully positioned but fail to get enough milk if his mother does not "let down" her milk. The let-down reflex occurs when oxytocin is released from your brain. As a result the breasts start to tingle and tense and the nipple stands out, and shortly afterward milk is ejected whether the baby is there or not. If this does not happen, the baby will only get a little of the thirst-quenching thin bluish foremilk and none of the richer, thicker hindmilk that contains more fat and satisfies the baby's hunger. The reflex can be inhibited if you are feeling self-conscious or nervous or if you are dreading a further assault on your nipples. It can help to visualize milk spurting out or to concentrate on something lovable about the baby. If other people are disturbing you, go elsewhere or ask them to leave. If you are afraid of feeding, try practicing relaxation and breathing techniques.

The length of time that a baby feeds is not as important as letting the baby take what he wants. He should feed for as long as he wants on one side and may not need the other breast at that feed. Babies vary enormously in their enthusiasm and efficiency in feeding, but they all get quicker with practice. The important thing to remember is that breastfeeding is an issue of supply and demand. The more often the baby demands milk by sucking on the breast, the greater the supply produced.

Your Position

Frequent feeding can put a considerable strain on your back if it is not well supported because the ligaments are still soft from the pregnancy and can be easily damaged. Ideally, you should sit in a chair with a high, straight back and arms. You may need a cushion behind your back, and while the baby is very small, you should place her on a pillow on your lap so that you do not have to bend over. Your back will ache badly if the baby is dragging on your breast as you feed or if you keep your head continually bent over and turned toward her. At night you may be able to feed while lying down in bed. The baby can be in any position that supports her and your back.

SORE NIPPLES

Even if the baby is well positioned, your nipples can become sore in the early days, which is hardly surprising when such a sensitive part of your body is suddenly subjected to intense wear. One study showed that 31 percent of first-time mothers who were breastfeeding had painful nipples on the fourth day after the birth of their baby. It also records considerable suffering with perineal pain and uterine cramps or afterpains, something that is often overlooked. Those conducting the trial found that mefenamic acid (Ponstan) was much more effective than acetaminophen at relieving postpartum pain.[2] Know that it does get better and that it is worth persevering. Your nipples can be acutely painful and even cracked, but they have the power to heal quite rapidly, as they get increasingly sensitive. There are numerous ways of helping yourself through this stage.

- Use a nipple shield made of latex or silicone. There are two types of nipple protector. One looks like a Mexican hat and acts as an extra layer of skin. The other has a rigid plastic casing with a teat on it, so that your milk is drawn out through the teat by suction alone, and there is no pressure on your nipple from the baby's mouth. You can buy them from a pharmacy. They have their disadvantages; it may take longer to feed, they need sterilizing between feeds, and if they are used for long the baby may reject the real thing. However, if used sparingly, while feeding from the nipple as often as possible, they can be invaluable. Research shows that use of nipple shields does not prevent successful breastfeeding.[3]

- Offer a pacifier. Some babies just enjoy sucking and would be quite content to stay at the breast all day. If your baby wants to nurse longer than you can stand, try offering a pacifier. Babies make it quite clear when they want food rather than comfort-sucking, and you can discard the pacifier at around three months without difficulty.

- Avoid letting your nipples get soggy with leaked milk. Try allowing a drop of milk to dry on the nipple, being topless and exposing the nipples to air and sunlight, or drying them with a hair dryer. Put a one-way diaper liner next to your skin with soft tissue paper behind it or make cages out of handleless metal tea strainers inserted into your bra. You could try sitting a foot away from a forty watt bulb with your nipples exposed to the heat several times a day.

- Try expressing milk by means of a pump (buy a syringe type or rent an electric one) and giving it to the baby in a bottle. This is a lot more work, but can provide a break which gives the nipple time to heal.

- Apply something to the nipple to help it heal, such as Hypercal, Calendula, Kamillosan, or vitamin E ointment. You could also try crushed cucumber or, if you are feeling strong, apply fresh lemon juice. This stings dreadfully at first, but really seems to work. A more soothing effect can be had by mixing slippery elm bark powder together with warm water and putting the paste between squares of muslin inside your bra. Another method of healing sore nipples is described in an Australian paper.[4] Midwives there have discovered that applying a geranium leaf—furry side to nipple—has been very successful in healing tender and cracked nipples.

Wash or wipe any preparation for soothing your nipples off them before you feed the baby.

- Anesthetize the nipple for the first few painful sucks by putting an ice cube on it before starting to feed. If the pain gets worse during the feed, the baby may not have latched correctly, and it could be worth breaking off and starting again.

Homeopathy

For simple soreness take Calendula internally, and also use the mother tincture externally. If the nipples are sore, cracked, and blistered, feel worse with warmth and at night, take Graphites. If the pain spreads from the nipple all over the body during feeding, if there are cracks especially on the right side, and if it feels worse with cold and damp, take Phytolacca.

NOT ENOUGH MILK

Even though you cannot completely empty a breast, there may be times when you feel that your baby is not getting enough. It is impossible to know exactly how much a breastfed baby is taking, but if the baby's diapers are wet, the stools soft and yellow, and he is gaining weight, then it is unlikely that the baby is not getting enough to eat overall. However, there are times when babies grow particularly fast and need more food, so that for a while you may feel that you do not have enough. The best remedy for insufficient milk is to keep on feeding. If you do that and do not short-circuit the demand-supply mechanism by giving complementary food, the supply should increase to match the baby's needs within a day or so.

If you are very active and do not eat adequately, you will find that your milk supply can start to fail. It is not indulgent to look after yourself when feeding, it is actually essential that you take some opportunity to rest, drink plenty of water, and eat three good meals plus snacks per day. If this seems a hopeless ideal, reflect that the baby depends on your well-being for its growth and physical and mental development.

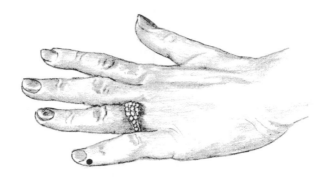

Acupressure point to increase the milk supply. Stimulate the point just below the nail on the side of your little finger with another nail or a matchstick.

This may make it easier to ask for help so that you can have at least one day's real rest.

There is a remedy that seems to work if you are really desperate to increase the milk supply. Known as "sugar shock," it involves taking a large amount of sugar, at least two heaped tablespoonfuls within one hour at the same time each day. It can be dissolved in lemon juice. It works by stimulating the pituitary gland and should be effective within a few days. If it has not worked within five days, abandon it.

Acupuncture

Consult an acupuncturist or try massaging the point just below the nail on the side of your little finger with another nail or a matchstick.

Aromatherapy

Mix two ounces of sweet almond oil with ten drops of fennel and ten drops of clary sage, and massage into your breasts. Wash it off before feeding.

Herbal Medicine

You can try drinking teas made from fennel, dill, anise, caraway, or cumin. Vervain, borage, and fenugreek are also noted for increasing your supply, while marshmallow, milkwort, and lettuce improve the quality. Some herbalists recommend chewing licorice root. Another suggestion is to take four tablespoons of brewer's yeast at lunch and suppertime or to try ten drops of alfalfa tincture in water, four times a day until the milk increases.

Homeopathy

In the absence of any other symptoms, Urtica urens is worth trying because it will rebalance the supply in whichever direction necessary; it is particularly useful if there is no milk at all. Use nettle tea until you get the remedy. For a weak flow right from the beginning, associated with anxiety, fatigue, and loss of sleep, use Causticum. If the milk slows down or stops, you are weak, pale, and maybe anemic, take Agnus castus. If the flow is very variable and changeable and you feel the same, try Pulsatilla. Additional causes may be: acute emotional experience, take Nat. mur.; sudden cold or damp, take Dulcemara or Pulsatilla; for sensitivity, if feeding causes unbearable sexual excitement, try Calc. phos.

ENGORGEMENT

Although your breasts will not stay engorged for more than a day or two at the start of breastfeeding, they can become engorged at any time thereafter if you have an unusually long interval between feeds, for instance if the baby sleeps longer than usual or is ill, or you are away from her. Whatever the cause, engorged breasts can be very uncomfortable indeed, and you may need to find some way of softening your breasts so that the baby can get the areola into her mouth. (It is important to wear a bra that will expand when your breasts are engorged because the swelling can add inches to your dimensions.)

The first remedy is to feed as often as possible and keep the breasts comfortable this way. You may need to express some milk first in order to soften the breast so that the baby can latch on, which is impossible if the breast is completely hard. This can be done by getting on your hands and knees in the bath or by leaning over a sink and splashing or spraying your breasts with warm water. This should help the milk to shoot out in threadlike jets.

You might prefer to save the milk for later on, because within a couple of weeks the supply will be adjusted to the baby's needs and it will be less abundant. You can express with a hand or electrical pump and store it in the freezer in small sterilized bottles. You can also catch the drips from the breast not in use in specially designed shells. It is important to freeze it straight after the feed so that the milk does not accumulate bacteria.

Other ways of helping to lessen the swelling include putting chilled cabbage leaves inside your bra and stroking the swelling from the nipple outward. You need to handle your breasts carefully because they can be easily bruised when they are engorged.

Aromatherapy

Either apply three drops of geranium oil in nonallergenic cream base or bathe the breasts with a lotion made up by adding six drops of geranium oil to one teaspoon (5 ml) of isopropyl alcohol or vodka and combining it with a pint (1 l) of water.

Too Much Milk

Although the problem of having too much milk does not cause anxiety, it can be very inconvenient to leak milk, flood the bed, and soak your clothes well past the early weeks. You can freeze the excess milk.

Aromatherapy

Add one drop of peppermint oil to a little water and soak two washcloths in it. Wrap around the breasts twice a day.

Herbal Medicine

If you really want to reduce the amount of milk you produce, try drinking teas of sage or herb robert *(Geranium robertianum)*.

Homeopathy

If you have too much milk, your breasts are hard and hot, and you are not thirsty, take one dose of Belladonna 6x hourly until there is an improvement.

BLOCKED DUCT OR MASTITIS

Sometimes one of the milk ducts in the breast may become blocked. It can happen if you wear clothes that constrict your breasts or if your arm presses on the breast. It results in pain in one specific area, which may become reddened and be tender and hard to the touch. If you do nothing about it, your temperature may rise and you will feel ill.

Start taking action at the first hint of tenderness or hardness. Encourage the baby to feed frequently on that side, and use a pump gently to express any remaining milk if it does not feel empty after feeding. While feeding or using the pump, stroke the hardened part toward the nipple—your partner can help with this—and vary the baby's position so that she is exerting the most suction on the blockage. Try having a hot bath and using a fine-toothed comb on your soapy breast to urge the lump out to your nipple. Swinging your arm around and around can improve the blood supply to the breast. Heather Welford, author of *A–Z of Feeding in the First Year*, suggests placing a hot water bottle wrapped in a towel next to the tender area if feeding is painful.

Aromatherapy

Try a compress of a drop each of rose, geranium, and lavender oils in one pint (500 ml) of cold water.

Herbal Medicine

You can take vitamin C (1 g) and six to eight garlic perles every three hours to combat infection or try two echinacea tablets every two hours. If you use the tincture use half a drop per pound of body weight per dose. Repeat the dose up to six times a day if you have a fever and continue taking it two to three times a day for seven days after the problem has eased.

If there is no improvement or you get worse, you may need antibiotics. There is no need to stop feeding, but remind your doctor that you are breastfeeding if he or she prescribes them. Take lactobacillus supplements with the antibiotics to prevent a subsequent yeast infection.

Homeopathy

If there is a sudden problem, take Aconite within the first twenty-four hours. If the breast is hard and perhaps hot, but the skin is not red, the breast is sensitive to touch and movement, and maybe worse on the left, take Bryonia. If the breast is hard, hot, red, painful, and extremely sensitive to touch and movement, and you feel restless, take Belladonna. If the pain is on the right and you are pale, not hot but are perspiring, try Calc. carb. When the breast is very hard and sensitive and is worse on the right, take Phytolacca. If an infection or abscess is indicated, as with a raised temperature and the problem is worse with warmth, worse at night and you are perspiring, try Mercurius. When there are hard lumps in the breast and you feel worse in the cold or damp, and the nipple may be retracted, use Silica. With stinging and burning, a cracked nipple, which is worse with the warmth of the bed and washing, and you crave fresh air, take Sulphur. If there are splinterlike pains, hypersensitivity and sweating and are much worse in the cold, take Hepar sulph.

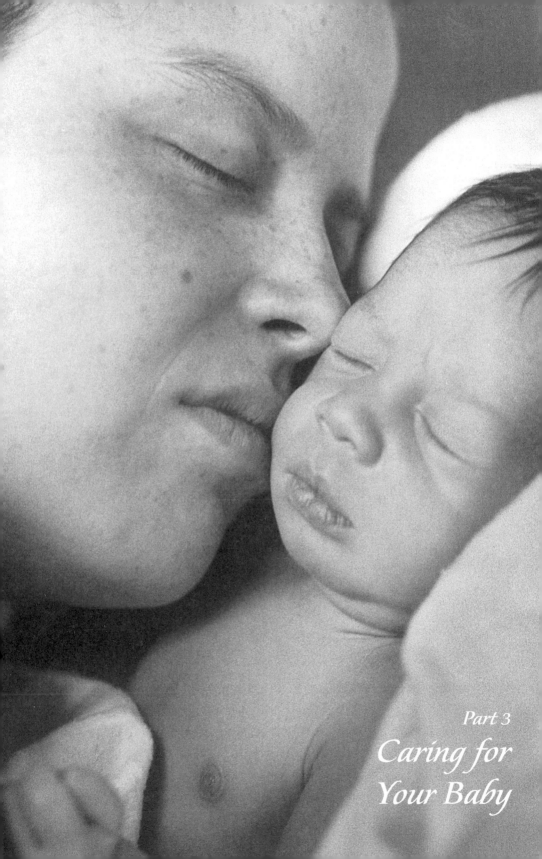

12

You and Your Baby

At some time after the birth—either hours or days—you will find yourself in charge of your new baby. This can be a moment of great triumph, but it may also be tempered with anxiety. Even if you are used to handling small babies, assuming full responsibility for your own can be daunting.

New parents are typically and understandably anxious about their new babies. They lack experience with that particular child, which is necessary for them to be able to feel confident about the way the baby is behaving. They are often unable to anticipate her needs, work out why she is crying, or have any idea of how she will behave in the next twenty-four hours. Babies are unpredictable and demanding, and although most will have settled down by the time they are three months old, the difficulties can seem overwhelming in those first few weeks of life.

Babies are in fact very tough and can survive quite considerable neglect, as demonstrated by the babies who lived for six days after the Mexican earthquake without any attention at all. In fact a certain amount of "neglect," such as that a second or subsequent child suffers by virtue of her place in the family, is healthy. However, it takes time for you to be that relaxed about your baby, and there are no short-cuts to gaining experience.

Make the most of the chance to absorb yourself in your first child because it will not come again. Remember, though, that you are not the only person in the world who can look after the baby, so accept offers of help and take the opportunity to go out or do something for your-self. It can be easy to feel that everything you do is connected with the baby—and children do take up an enormous part of every day—and this can cause an undercurrent of resentment. It is quite normal to feel that you as an individual are being lost, that your interests are over-looked, and that you are now only X's mother. Again, this should only be a brief stage, but handing the baby over from time to time can make it seem much briefer.

CARE OF THE UMBILICUS

The cord will have been cut and clamped with string, elastic, or a plastic clamp. The clamp is released after a few hours, and then it is a matter of a few days before the stump of the cord dries up and drops off. Because there is a risk of the umbilicus becoming infected (greater in a hospital), the stump is usually swabbed with alcohol and dusted with anti-staphylococcal powder. Some midwives have discovered that it heals best and the cord comes off most quickly if it is cleaned with water alone, and the baby is bathed frequently.

Alternatively, you can dress the stump with honey, which is a natural antiseptic, or dry it up with witch hazel. Calendula powder is useful for healing. It is important to prevent the diaper from irritating the stump while it is healing. Your midwife will not discharge the baby from her care until the stump falls off.

JAUNDICE IN NEW BABIES

Some jaundice is very common in new babies and shows itself by turning the baby's skin and the white of the eyes yellow, often giving the baby the appearance of a healthy tan. Usually jaundice starts between the second and third day, and it is caused when the liver breaks down the extra red blood cells that are no longer needed once the baby is breathing and taking in his own oxygen. The cells are broken down and converted into, among other products, bilirubin, which is fat soluble and needs to be made water soluble so that it can be excreted. If this does not occur, the bilirubin remains and gathers in fatty tissue under the skin, staining it yellow, and around the kidneys. Occasionally, it collects around the basal ganglia of the brain, and this can lead to kernicterus if jaundice is not treated, a condition that causes brain damage. If the baby's color deepens and he seems lethargic, blood will be taken to ensure that bilirubin levels are not rising too high.

Orthodox treatment consists of putting the baby under special lights. You can try a home version by exposing the baby to natural sunlight by putting his crib under the window. Jaundice is more common in babies whose mothers have been given synthetic oxytocin and ergometrine or pitocin.

Alternative remedies include drinking at least two cups of catnip or dandelion tea daily, and giving Nat. phos. tissue salt 6x to the baby.

Another suggestion is to give the baby molasses water (one teaspoon molasses to one cup of cooled boiled water) by dropper after each feed until the milk comes in.

SLEEP

In the early weeks the baby cannot be expected to sleep according to any particular pattern or recognize night from day, although some do. Sometimes you will find that the baby has periods of activity at the same time as before birth.

One way to encourage sleep at night is to make it clear to the baby that it is not a playtime. Feed the baby when necessary and change her if essential, but don't talk to or play with her. Keep the light down, and put the baby back into her crib as soon as possible. If she is cold, put a hot water bottle in the crib when you take her out, so that it is warm when you put her back. Playing a long-playing musical box after a feeding so that the baby comes to associate the sound with going to sleep is sometimes effective. Alternately, a tape of uterine sounds may help both of you to get back to sleep after being woken. Having the baby's crib beside your bed means that you can feed her without fully waking.

A few babies sleep through the night by the time they are six weeks old, but most do not and may not for many months yet. Creating a routine can help, and there is a case for saying that if you do not respond to night crying for food, the baby will stop demanding it within a week. This is only recommended for babies of twelve pounds (6 kg) or more and is hard to do, although it does seem to work.

Many mothers end up with the baby sleeping in the bed beside them. A recent, large survey showed that as many as 50 percent of parents slept with their baby in the bed when the baby was six months old. Provided that you are not under the influence of drugs or alcohol, the baby will be safe.

As with everything else, babies vary in their need for sleep, some being almost permanently asleep and others hardly ever shutting their eyes. A nonsleeper is harder work because you get much less chance to sleep or do anything for yourself. A baby like this may develop into the type of adult that needs little sleep, but the problem can also be caused by allergy (see pages 173–174) or the torsion on the brain caused by the pressures exerted at birth. In this case, cranial osteopathy can work brilliantly so that a child may start sleeping normally within a day of the treatment.

Avena sativa compound, which is a combination of oats, hops, passion flower, and valerian, can be taken by mothers and children. It is said to be a natural aid to peaceful relaxation and particularly useful after a stressful day. To aid sleep take ten to twenty drops in a little water a half hour before retiring. Repeat the dose if necessary. Children should be given half the adult dose.

Acupressure may also work well; an acupuncturist will show you the technique of rubbing the acupuncture points relevant to your baby.

Baby massage given an hour or two before expected periods of restlessness or sleeplessness may help to soothe the baby and improve the problem. You can find out how best to do it by taking the baby to someone who specializes in baby massage or consulting the books mentioned in the suggested reading list. Recently published research presented by Dr. Elvidina Adamson-Macedo of Britain's Wolverhampton University shows that premature babies who were stroked for twenty minutes a day for three weeks were better at intelligence tests, reading, and comprehension when tested at the age of seven than a control group. They were also assessed as being healthier. It is thought that stroking increases the level of endorphins, natural relaxants and painkillers, which then strengthened the children's immune systems.[1]

Massage techniques for use on premature babies have evolved but are equally applicable for full-term babies.[2] They include the following suggestions.

- Before beginning, make sure your hands are warm, turn on heat source, undress the baby if necessary, and lay her on a towel in whichever position you have chosen, keeping a diaper at hand. You can use a cornstarch-based baby powder sprinkled onto your hands (make sure your baby does not inhale it) or use oil. A good baby massage oil is made by mixing one ounce of sweet almond oil with two drops of rose.
- With the baby lying on her back, facing you, begin at the head and apply butterfly-light effleurage (superficial stroking) strokes from the back of the head to the front, using each hand in turn.
- Gradually make the strokes wider and wider to take in the sides of the head, the ears, and the neck, repeating the motion as often as you like, making the strokes firmer as you get used to the feel of the baby.
- Gradually make the strokes wider so that you can glide all the way down the chest and abdomen. The abdomen may be stroked in a circular motion, particularly good for windy babies because

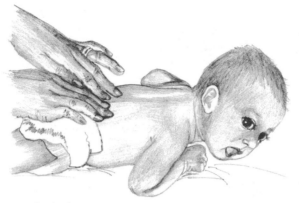

Back massage for baby.

it helps digestion. Next, clasp the arms and legs in turn, gently separate the toes and fingers and squeeze lightly, talking to the baby all the while.

• Now lie the baby on her front, and using the same method as for the chest and abdomen, apply light effleurage strokes from the shoulder blades to the buttocks, this time incorporating small circular movements all along the spine. This completes the massage. For premature babies this massage is recommended every four to six hours, when the baby is either not hungry or has been fed recently.

It is best to avoid sedating the baby because the drugs often work in reverse, making the baby even more active and less likely to sleep. With a toddler patterns of sleeplessness can often be broken by sending the child to spend the night with relatives or friends.

WEANING

You need not start weaning your breastfed baby until he is at least six months old, providing that you are eating well and the baby is gaining weight. Growth spurts occur at around three weeks, six weeks, and three months, and the increased demand at these times may make you feel that you are not providing enough milk and query the need for solid food. If you keep breastfeeding, the milk supply will increase within forty-eight hours, although in the meantime the baby may seem hungry and wake more often.

When you start introducing solid foods, it is best to introduce one food at a time and delay the introduction of milk, wheat, and eggs. If you have a family history of allergies or if the baby has shown any hint of an allergic response, such as colic, eczema, or asthma, you might want to start him on the following weaning diet suggested by Dr. Andrew Cant (of the Royal Victoria Newcastle Hospital) and Janet Bailes (of St. George's Hospital, London).

Start by introducing food in the order given below, offering it daily for a week, and watching carefully to see if it causes a skin rash or loose, watery stools. If there is a reaction avoid the food for several months.

1. Milk-free baby rice (check the label on the box) mixed with water or expressed breast milk.
2. Puréed root vegetables, such as potatoes, carrots, parsnips, rutabagas, turnips.
3. Puréed fruit, such as apple, pear, banana, but no citrus fruits until the baby is nine months old.
4. Other vegetables, such as peas, beans, lentils, broccoli, etc.
5. Other cereals, but no wheat until the baby is eight months old.
6. Lamb, turkey, and then the other meats.
7. Fish, but not until ten months.
8. Other milk and milk products, but not before ten months. If the baby is having less than four feeds a day, you may need to give soy milk. Start with yogurt, boiled cow's milk, and then if these are tolerated, introduce cheese, butter, etc.
9. Eggs, but not until one year.

13

Illness in Babies

As you get to know your child, you will develop the intuition that tells you when he is not well, and whether the illness is serious or not. At first, however, you will not know your baby's individual behavior patterns well enough to do this, and babies behave unpredictably even when perfectly well, so that in the early days you are likely to have lots of worries about his health. This is not necessarily a bad thing; some degree of anxiety is useful and even experienced mothers feel the need for extra caution with their new babies.

Illness in babies is a bit like labor—you can be certain if it is the real thing, but it is less easy to be sure if it only might be. When the child is older you will know what you can treat yourself and what requires medical attention, but in the meantime the following symptoms should alert you to the presence of a serious illness:

- Fits, convulsions, not breathing, unconsciousness.
- Difficulty in breathing, grunting, rapid breathing.
- Skin blue or very pale.

- Unexplained bleeding from any part of the body.
- Stiff neck and irritability.
- Rash that does not fade when pressed on with a clear drinking glass.

Signs of Illness

Watch out for these signs of illness and seek medical help when necessary.

- The child is unusually hot or cold (test by kissing her forehead). Bear in mind that young babies can be quite ill with a normal or lowered temperature. A raised temperature may mean that the hands and feet are cold while the forehead is hot. If the baby's temperature is high, take any clothes off and keep the child cool by sponging with tepid water or using a fan if the temperature rises above 102°F (39.4°C).
- The baby refuses more than one feed or meal.
- A blocked nose prevents the baby from feeding.
- Continual or unusual screaming or crying.
- The child is obviously in pain.
- Frequent vomiting or diarrhea. This is particularly serious in babies and children because they can quickly become dehydrated.
- The child refuses to smile. A child can sound very ill with a hacking cough but be all right if she is able to smile, eat, and play. A sick child gives all these things up and is either very fretful and unhappy or spends a lot of time sleeping.

If you take your child to a doctor, there are certain questions you should ask about your child's illness.

1. What is the diagnosis? This can be useful to know for the future. However, often there is not any positive diagnosis, just that the child is ill but not seriously and will probably get better without treatment.
2. What is the treatment? Not all childhood illnesses require antibi-

otics, but if you are given medicines take notes of the dosage and common side effects. Ask about alternatives too.

3. How soon will it be before the child is likely to improve?
4. Are there any signs you should look out for that might suggest the child is getting worse?
5. When should you bring the child back if there is no improvement?
6. How long is the child likely to be infectious (if applicable)?

Trust your instinct and be persistent if you think there is something really wrong.

WHEN TO CALL THE DOCTOR

Word of mouth is the best way of finding a good doctor. Ask other mothers whom they recommend. Some doctors are happy to talk to you before you make an appointment. Doctors who have young children themselves may be the most sympathetic and understanding. You need to:

- Check that you can consult your doctor by phone.
- Be sure that they answer night calls themselves.
- Ensure that they will see a sick child the same day in their office.

It is usually safe to take a child with a fever to the doctor's office by car, although you should let the receptionist know if you think your child is infectious. Put your baby in clothes that undo easily and take a spare diaper.

If you have difficulty in deciding whether to call the doctor—and it is usually in the early hours of the morning that this seems to be the greatest problem—consider how you would advise a friend in the same situation, or if you would drive the child to a hospital or drive miles to an open drugstore if necessary. A good doctor would rather you called unnecessarily than fail to call when you think that something is wrong. If your child is suddenly and seriously ill or has a bad accident, call an ambulance or take him to the nearest emergency room. Make sure you know how to get there before you need it.

First Aid

Small babies tend to have fewer accidents than children, although there is a first time for each advance they make, as many a mother discovers when her baby rolls off the changing mat. However they soon grow into an extremely accident-prone phase, where you have to anticipate their every move.

There are some alternative remedies that work incredibly well and are well worth keeping in a first aid box for the inevitable accident. Arnica or a combination of Aconite, Belladonna, and Chamomilla, often called ABC tablets, administered after any serious fall or bang are very effective, and both you and the child may benefit from Rescue Remedy after an accident. Take four drops of the remedy in water or drop directly into the mouth. Nelson–Bach, a manufacturer of homeopathic remedies, offers a range of creams or ointments that provide rapid and effective treatment for a number of minor ailments, including Arnica cream for bruising. Applied immediately, the treatment removes the pain and stops the bruise from developing (avoid applying to broken skin). For burns hold the area that has been burned or scalded under cold running water for ten minutes, and then apply the ointment all over and around the area. This eases the pain and prevents blistering. Hypercal (hypericum and calendula) ointment is good for healing cuts and sores and can be very good for skin complaints. There is also a pyrethrum spray for bites and stings that is very effective.

Infectious Diseases

Babies may be less likely to pick up the common childhood diseases because they retain a certain immunity from their mothers for the first six months or so. This may mean that if they do come into prolonged contact with a disease because an older brother or sister has it, they may only get it very mildly. Some diseases such as whooping cough and measles can be very serious in babies who are too young to be immunized against them, so it is very important to make sure you avoid contact with known cases.

Rubella (German Measles)

Incubation period ranges from fourteen to twenty-one days. It starts as a flat pink rash beginning behind the ears and giving rise to enlarged glands at the back of the neck. This disease is generally mild, but keep away from pregnant women who have not been immunized. This is only likely to apply to first pregnancies as nonimmune women are usually immunized after birth. Blood is tested for immune status when you start prenatal care.

Measles

Incubation period ranges from ten to fifteen days. Starts as a bad cold with a cough and red eyes and perhaps a fever. Look for white spots on the inside of the cheeks. After a few days dark red spots cover the body, and the child develops a high fever, may have no appetite, and seems very ill. There can be complications of bronchitis, ear infections, and, more rarely, inflammation of the brain. The child is no longer infectious once the symptoms are gone. A homeopathic prophylaxis, preventing the child from contracting the disease, is to give Pulsatilla 30x daily from the third day after contact until the fifteenth or sixteenth day, when the danger of infection will have passed. If measles develops, contact a homeopath although you may find Bryonia helpful generally, and Euphrasia should help inflamed eyes and eyelids. See pages 189 to 190 about treating the high fever that often accompanies measles. A bath including four drops of eucalyptus may ease the spots.

Whooping Cough

Incubation period is from seven to ten days. Starts as a cough and cold and then develops the typical whoop although this may not be present in babies. The cough takes the child by surprise so that they are forced to cough before taking a breath. Each prolonged cough may end in vomiting. Whooping cough is said to be noninfectious twenty-eight days from the start of symptoms, but the cough may last longer. A homeopathic prophylaxis is to give your baby three doses of Pertussin 30x at any time after it is six months old. Give one dose one night, one the following morning, and then one that night. If the child is in contact with whooping cough, give one dose of Pertussin 30x once a week for three weeks. It should only be given to babies under three months in consultation with a homeopath.

If the child does get whooping cough, seek help from a homeopath. The following remedies should prove helpful. Give Drosera for whooping cough with spasms of coughing that follow on top of each other and result in gagging and vomiting, or if the cough is worse at night and when the child lies down. For a suffocating cough that makes the child stiff and blue in the face and results in vomiting of phlegm, give Ipecac. Consult a homeopathic pharmacy about the use of Pertuderon 1x and 11x, which can be very helpful in alleviating symptoms.

Chicken Pox

Incubation period is about fourteen days. Starts with spots that soon become clear blisters that become pustules and soon turn into scabs. Not a particularly serious illness but can cause severe itching. It is no longer infectious once the spots have turned to scabs.

To prevent itching, add four drops of peppermint, tea tree, or eucalyptus oil to a bath, and dab spots with diluted distilled witch hazel, or calamine lotion. Hypercal cream applied to the spots before they blister seems to make them less severe.

Mumps

Incubation period is about twenty-one days. Starts with the gland in front of the ear swelling and becoming tender. One or both sides may be affected. The child may have difficulty in drinking and eating. The child is infectious for seven days after the swelling has gone down.

Tetanus

Homeopathic prophylaxis (need not be given in the first year unless you live in the country) consists of two doses of Hypericum 200x per week for one month.

Diphtheria

This is very rare nowadays, but you can protect your child from the disease by giving Diphtherium 30x once a week for four to six weeks.

IMMUNIZATION

This is a controversial issue about which you will have to make up your own mind after inquiring about all the facts both for and against. It is a decision that parents often agonize about. Some homeopaths believe that fighting the common childhood illnesses with immunization makes the child weaker by suppressing the immune system.

If you decide not to have your child immunized, you may want to ask a homeopath about prophylactic remedies in an epidemic. If your child does contract one of the diseases, it can be treated homeopathically to reduce its length and strength, for example whooping cough treated homeopathically lasts only seven days.

If you do choose to immunize, the ill effects can be minimized by giving Arnica or Thuja 30x beforehand.

14

An A~Z of Common Infant Complaints and Their Remedies

ALLERGIES

There seems to be an increase in the number of babies and children experiencing allergic reactions to either their food or something in their environment. You might suspect allergy if your baby is unusually fretful, has diarrhea or constipation, is particularly thirsty, sleeps little or fitfully, has a body rash (see remedies for eczema, page 188) or frequent diaper rash (see pages 186–187), is colicky (see pages 178–182), seems to have a perpetual cold, has dark rings under the eyes or has puffy swelling around them, or a bloated abdomen.

Very susceptible babies (those with one or both parents with an allergy themselves) can react to minute traces of your food in your breast milk. They may react very badly to formula (see diet for weaning, page 163). Fruit juices and vitamin drops can also cause problems. It can help to identify the cause if you make a chart of the baby's food intake and subsequent responses.

Babies can also react to the things in contact with their skin. This might be wool or the laundry detergent or fabric softener used in washing clothes and bedding (see remedies for diaper rash, pages 186–187); or it could be the soap, baby bath liquid, shampoo, lotion, or wipes used in cleaning the baby. Eliminate the cause and wash the baby with water alone, or ask your doctor to prescribe Oilatum, a liquid emulsion that is put into bath water and cleans without irritating the skin.

Wheezy babies may be reacting to the house dust mite that lives in dust and bedding. If your child is unlucky enough to suffer from this allergy, you may find the condition improves with scrupulous attention to damp dusting and daily vacuuming, although some have found vacuuming to exacerbate the allergy.

Allergic children should be under the supervision of a doctor, although they are not all open-minded about the diagnosis. Food-allergic children should be seen by a dietician; your doctor can refer you to a community dietician.

You may want to consider eating a low-allergen diet yourself if you are pregnant and think your baby is likely to be allergic to food. There is no real evidence yet that this will prevent the baby from acquiring allergies, but it is thought to help. You will need dietary advice.

Eliminating the cause of the problem may be sufficient to ensure your child's health but also consider constitutional treatment from a homeopath for you or the baby. Acupressure can have a dramatic effect on allergic children, reducing the sensitivity overnight, and reflexology can work well too.

ASTHMA

This may start as a nocturnal cough and frequent colds. You should have it diagnosed by a medical practitioner, but you can have it treated by a homeopath, osteopath, or reflexologist. Asthma is more likely in children whose parents smoke and those who are bottle-fed.

Burns

See section on first aid, page 168. If the burns are severe, give Cantharis to prevent infection.

Chest Infections

Babies can have horrible-sounding coughs and yet not be seriously ill. Sometimes, though, the cough may not sound particularly bad, but the infection will have traveled down the respiratory tract so that it is described as being "in the chest" and therefore potentially more serious. It can be hard to decide by yourself if this has occurred, although you can listen to your baby's chest without a stethoscope by putting your ear to her chest or back. It is a good idea to have babies with a cough checked medically, although older children are unlikely to be ill this way without a fever or seeming sick in other ways.

Sometimes a chest infection leads to breathing difficulties such as wheezing, being unable to inhale enough air or to exhale, and breathing much faster than forty breaths a minute, which may result in the baby turning blue or the lower ribs or the skin at the neck being sucked in. Any of these signs are an indication for seeking immediate help.

Frequent night coughs and attacks of wheezy bronchitis may be an indication of asthma (see page 174) in susceptible children.

Herbal Medicine

Breastfed babies can be treated for infection through their mothers. Echinacea is an effective antimicrobial herb, which works for both viruses and bacteria. Use one to two teaspoonfuls of the root in a cupful of water, simmered for fifteen minutes. Drink three times a day. Maintain the treatment for at least seven days, even when the condition is improved.

Homeopathy

Give ABC tablets, a combination of Aconite, Belladonna, and Chamomilla, which are useful at the start of any childhood illness. For a dry painful cough, try Bryonia. For a barking cough or a constant tickling cough, try Drosera. For a cough with coarseness and loss of voice, try Phosphorus.

CHOKING

It is terrifying to find your child choking and turning blue from lack of breath. Make sure you know what to do in case it happens. First, call for medical help. If the problem is caused by food obstructing the airway, or by fluid having been inhaled, try the following procedures.

If the child is less than one year old, hold the child upside down and clap the back between the shoulder blades five times. Then, with two fingers pressed into the child's chest, centered between the nipples, thrust upward five times.

For the child over one year old, use the Heimlich maneuver. With child sitting upright or on your knee, wrap your arms around the child from behind, make a fist with one hand, and place it thumbside in, at a point on the abdomen just above the navel and below the rib cage. Then press quickly upward as before. The upward pressure of air below the obstruction should force it out.

This type of resuscitation can also be done if the child becomes unconscious. Lie the child down face upward. Put one hand on the child's abdomen so that the heel of it is on the spot just above the navel and below the rib cage. Put your other hand over the first one. Then push the abdomen with a quick upward thrust and repeat as necessary. For more information on first-aid techniques, contact your local chapter of the American Red Cross.

Take Rescue Remedy yourself for shock afterward and give it or Aconite to the child. If the child is bruised by the procedure, give Arnica.

COLDS

The more babies are exposed to other people, the greater the likelihood of them picking up a cold or cough, even when very small. Babies with

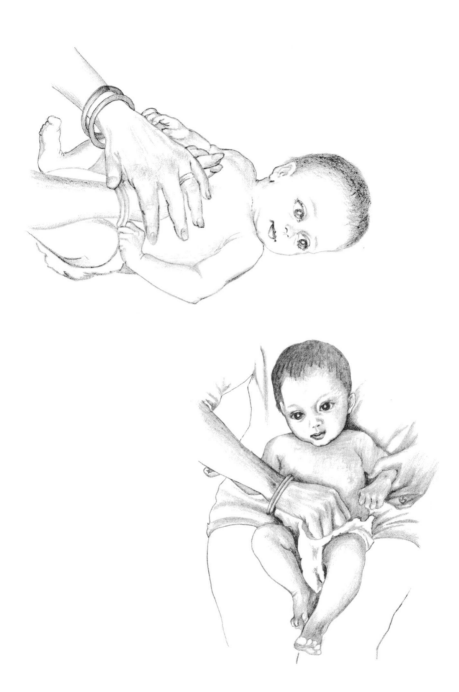

The Heimlich maneuver. Performed on a child (top) face upward; (bottom) sitting upright.

older brothers or sisters will be exposed to them from the start. You will feel happier if people with obvious colds keep away from your new baby, but it is unrealistic to isolate your baby totally, so your baby is likely to get one sometime.

Colds in babies often last two weeks or more, and can seem to be continual during the winter. In most cases the child is fretful and may wake more often and have problems feeding but is not seriously ill.

You can help a baby with a blocked nose to feed by removing the mucus with a dropper or bulb syringe. Decongestant drops can help, but they must be used sparingly as they become ineffective within a few days. You can also make breathing easier by rubbing Vick's ointment on the chest or by putting a drop of eucalyptus oil on the sheet at the head end of the bed.

Central heating can make things worse by drying the atmosphere. You can increase the humidity by putting wet towels over the radiators or using a humidifier.

If your child always has a streaming nose, it would be worth thinking about whether the cause was not in fact a cold, but an allergy (see pages 173–174). Colds can cause real problems if they result in middle ear or chest infections (see page 175).

Homeopathy

Give Aconite two or three times on the first day of a cold. For a sneezy cold with a nose running like a tap, try Nat. mur. For flulike colds, try Gelsemium. For a feverish head cold, try Merc. sol.

COLIC

Colic is a horrible problem that sometimes afflicts small babies. It can start at any time after birth and typically lasts for three months. It can strike at any time of the day or night and often occurs at the same time each evening. It causes the baby to start crying suddenly and with a desperate intensity, giving every appearance of being in acute pain. It often comes in spasms that make the baby arch his back or draw his knees up to his chest. The attacks can last an hour or more, and subside gradually leaving the baby and parents exhausted. It can be agonizing to see your tiny baby in agony and be unable to help him. You start by feeling deeply sorry for the infant, but as the crying continues you can become maddened and would do anything to stop it.

Colic does usually pass with time, and it does not appear to do the baby any lasting damage. Its causes are not fully understood, although it does seem to be connected with the immaturity of the baby's digestive system. It often ends as abruptly as it started at around thirteen weeks. You can just sit it out or try some of the following remedies, although it is possible that only time will help. There are lots of suggested remedies, perhaps reflecting the degree of despair to which colic can drive parents.

During an attack, the baby may be calmed by being held over the shoulder and walked around. A pacifier can be a godsend even if you have to hold it in, because the sucking instinct will sometimes win over the need to cry. Some babies feel better if they are held on your lap on their tummies, and heat from a warm hot water bottle (not hot) on the tummy helps too. A tape of uterine sounds played loudly near the baby's head can make a great difference, and some people think that giving a spoonful of boiled water before a feeding helps. You may find that adding Rescue Remedy to the water makes a considerable difference.

The colic may be cured or lessened by a change in the baby's milk. Many colicky babies are allergic to either their formula milk or some constituent of their mother's breast milk. A bottle-fed baby may be better on soy milk, and a breastfed baby may improve if you give up eating possible allergens, especially milk and eggs. This is because tiny particles of these proteins are present in your milk as little as two hours after eating them, and sensitive babies may react to them with colic or eczema, diarrhea, and vomiting.

If you are breastfeeding and restricting your diet for longer than a week, you will have to make sure that you do not suffer from a lack of balance in your diet. Your doctor can refer you to a dietician. Try eliminating the following common allergens from your diet for a week. If there is no improvement, do not continue with it, but if there is, start by introducing the foods singly, leaving at least two days between each kind, so that you can monitor the baby's reaction. You *must* be scrupulous about excluding the forbidden foods.

- Milk in any form, i.e., butter, cheese, cream, yogurt, skimmed milk powder (can also be found in processed food as sodium caseinate, caseinate, whey, or nonfat milk solids).
- Eggs (also yolk, white, lactalbumin, and egg lecithin).
- Wheat, including bread and any of the many products that include wheat flour.
- Chocolate and cocoa, even milk-free.
- Citrus fruits and tomatoes.
- Beef and poultry.
- Any other food or drink that seems to give your baby colic. It may help to keep a food diary and a chart of the crying spells.

If the baby does respond to dietary measures, it might be wise to delay weaning as long as possible and to avoid the above foods when you do start (see pages 162–163).

Acupuncture

An acupuncturist can help improve your baby's colic. You may be able to help yourself by exerting pressure between the baby's first and second toes at a point a finger's breadth from the base. This will calm the liver, relax the muscles, and reduce inflammation.

Aromatherapy

Try dipping a small towel in warm water to which a few drops of chamomile oil have been added, wringing it out, and placing it over the baby's stomach.

Finally, you will need help and support through this troubled time. Your midwife, doctor, or other mothers may be able to give you practical support.

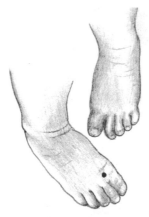

Acupressure point for easing colic. Exert pressure between the baby's first and second toes at a point a finger's breadth from the base.

Cranial Osteopathy

This can help some babies by freeing the cranial base and relieving distortions of the skull that may be causing pressure on the vagus nerve leading to gastric irritation.

Mohammed had cried almost from the moment of his forceps birth. He had bad attacks of colic lasting up to an hour after almost every feed, and at six weeks his parents were getting desperate. He was taken to a cranial osteopath who treated him for about forty minutes. He seemed to enjoy the treatment, settling down and going to sleep. He released a lot of wind from his bowel and seemed calmer when he woke up. He went back for further treatments and gradually the colic improved.

Herbal Medicine

The remedies can be passed through the breast milk or given directly to the baby. You can drink decoctions of dill, fennel, or the bruised seeds of aniseed, or eat coriander leaves or ginger, either fresh or cooked. You could give the baby a teaspoonful of dill, catnip, or chamomile tea.

Homeopathy

It is preferable for a baby suffering from colic to be seen by a trained homeopath so that an individual diagnosis and treatment can be made.

Massage

There are particular techniques of massage to help babies with colic and other problems. Regular massage is considered beneficial for all babies. You can find out about the techniques by reading the booklet *Massage for Life* by Stephen Russell and Yehudi Gordon.

CONSTIPATION

This is only a problem if passing infrequent stools causes the baby distress. Some breastfed babies go for days without a bowel movement, and it causes them no discomfort. Bottle-fed babies are more likely to have bulky, hard stools that can be difficult to pass. If you think the baby needs some help because she is uncomfortable, you could give her some diluted prune juice or try taking syrup of figs or eat prunes or figs yourself if breastfeeding.

Homeopathy

If the rectum is inactive so that the baby has to strain to pass a soft stool and can only do so when there is a large accumulation, give Alumina. If the problem persists, consult a homeopath.

Massage

Massage can relieve constipation and also works for colic, indigestion, vomiting, and diarrhea. Stephen Russell recommends a series of Taoist massage patterns in *Massage for Life*. This one, known as Harmonizing Fire and Water is the first of eight patterns that are good for releasing tensions in the abdomen. This should be done preferably at a quiet time and with the baby naked.

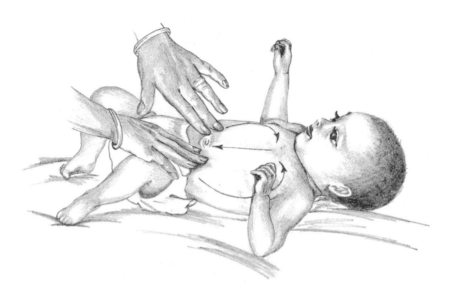

Baby massage for colic, constipation, indigestion, vomiting, and diarrhea.

Using as much pressure as would smooth a crumpled piece of tissue paper without tearing it, stroke the baby. Start at the midline of the chest using the fingers of both hands, move down the torso to the pubic bone, then separate the hands to the sides of the torso, and pull up into the armpits. Circle over the breast region and meet again on the midline at the chest. This balances the heart and the kidneys. Do this for up to twenty-one cycles, each lasting ten seconds. Massage with great sensitivity and delicacy to achieve the best results. It builds physical and emotional stability, helps to calm a hyperactive child, relaxes the chest, and strengthens the digestive system.

CRADLE CAP

This is a kind of thick, scaly dandruff that often forms on the scalp and eyebrows of babies. To get rid of it, dab the affected area with olive oil (not baby oil, which is mineral oil and can damage the skin), allow the scales to soften for a couple of hours or longer, and then rub firmly with a rough dry towel. Shampoo and dry the hair.

CROUP

This is an acute inflammation of the vocal cords, which results in a frightening attack of breathing difficulties, usually in the middle of the night. The child goes to bed with a slight cold, maybe sounding a little hoarse and wakes up in the early hours with a distinctive harsh cough and difficulty in sucking in enough air. Your child is likely to be terrified—and so are you—but it is important not to show it.

Humidity helps so boil an electric kettle continuously in the bedroom or use a humidifier to fill the air with steam. You can make a tent with sheets to concentrate the steam as long as you are careful. Hold and comfort your child, and there should be an improvement within fifteen minutes so that you can all go back to bed.

If there is no improvement or if the condition seems to be getting worse and the child cannot settle or has a high temperature or you are really worried, take the child to a hospital where he can be put into an oxygen tent.

Herbal Medicine

Give thirty drops of bloodroot tincture.

Homeopathy

Give Aconite for fear, and take it yourself. Then give Spongia or Hepar sulph.

DIAPER RASH

Most babies get diaper rash at some time. It is easier to prevent than to cure. It starts for all sorts of reasons, including a reaction to something on the skin—this may be anything from the lotion, soap and water, cream, disposable wipes, or even the diaper. If you are using cloth diapers, the baby can be sensitive to the laundry detergent or fabric softener. Use a pure soap washing powder and cut out the fabric softener, and put diapers through an extra rinse cycle. Some mothers find that changing the brand of disposable diapers cures the rash.

Diaper rash is sometimes caused by teething or by food the child has eaten—fruit juice, for instance, often causes a rash. To cope with it, change the diaper more frequently and use one of the healing ointments, such as calendula, Hypercal, chickweed, or comfrey. Nelson–Bach's ointment for burns may help.

Aromatherapy

Add a drop of tea tree oil to diaper cream.

Herbal Medicine

You can try mixing up a paste of goldenseal and slippery elm bark powder with water and putting it onto the skin. If possible leave the diaper off altogether for as long as possible or put on oversized diapers to allow air to the baby's bottom.

If the rash forms in patches or islands, it may be caused by thrush. Treat this with an anitfungal cream from the doctor, or make an ointment by adding a handful of the herb thuja to seven ounces (200 g) of Vaseline, simmering it for ten minutes, then straining it through fine gauze, pressing out the liquid. Pour into a container and seal.

You may find that lightly whipping egg white and dabbing it onto the skin at changing time for twenty-four hours may clear the rash up. A commercial diaper-rash ointment spread very thinly over the bottom can also be very useful.

Homeopathy

Give a combination of the three tissue salts Nat. phos., Nat. sulph., and Nat. silica to correct any acid or alkaline imbalance. Where the skin is red, very hot, and flaky, give Arsen. alb.

Diarrhea

This is unusual in breastfed babies, who normally have several seedy, yellow, fluid stools per day. Suspect diarrhea if the stools become unusually watery, frequent, or smell different. It is more common in bottle-fed babies because formula does not have the same protective qualities as breast milk. Alternating between the two can lead to diarrhea by altering the pH balance in the gut.

Diarrhea must be taken seriously in babies because they do not have to lose much fluid to become seriously dehydrated. Dehydration is indicated if the baby's eyes are sunken, the soft spot on the top of its head becomes concave, and the skin is losing its elasticity. In this case you will be able to pinch a fold of skin, and it will take far longer than usual to return to normal. The baby's mouth will be dry, and the urine output will be scanty and dark yellow. If any of these symptoms is present, call your doctor.

Remedies for mild diarrhea include giving the baby a teaspoonful of puréed carrot, giving one ounce (25 ml) of the water in which rice has been boiled, or maintaining the balance of electrolytes by giving the baby boiled water and Pedialyte, a salt and dextrose mixture available from the drugstore. In an emergency make your own with one pint ($1/2$ liter) boiled water, one tablespoonful sugar, honey or glucose, one-eighth teaspoon sodium bicarbonate and one-eighth teaspoon salt. Persistent diarrhea can be caused by allergy (see page 173). Baby massage can help.

Diarrhea can cause awful diaper rash, so be sure to change the diaper as soon as it is dirtied, and put lots of cream on to protect the skin from acid stools.

Toddler diarrhea, known as "peas and carrots syndrome," results in chronic diarrhea with the food passing through the child only partially digested, and often follows an attack of gastroenteritis. Small doses of a milk-free form of lactobacillus may help as well.

Herbal Medicine

A little yarrow or meadowsweet decoction may ease the problem.

Homeopathy

Give ABC at the start. For diarrhea with or without vomiting, from food that was bad, or from too much fruit—give Arsen. alb. every two hours. If it persists, consult a homeopath. For painless diarrhea give Acid. phos. For green slimy stools during teething, give Chamomilla.

EAR INFECTIONS

A cold can lead to an infection of the middle ear, which causes the eardrum to bulge out painfully. Although the cause may not be immediately apparent, you will know that something is wrong if your baby has earache, because she is likely to cry a lot, put her hand to her ear if old enough, and may develop a temperature. If it is left untreated, the pus will eventually build up so that the eardrum bursts and the pus drains out. Although the eardrum is likely to heal satisfactorily, many doctors prefer to treat the condition with antibiotics to avoid the slight risk of the infection spreading and to stop the pain. Some children suffer repeatedly from ear infections and can be helped by treatment from a cranial osteopath, homeopath, or reflexologist.

Aromatherapy

Maggie Tisserand suggests putting one drop of lavender oil on a cotton ball and gently inserting it in the child's outer ear to ease the pain.

Homeopathy

Give ABC at the first sign of earache. If the child is changeable, pathetic, and not thirsty, give Pulsatilla 30x. If the earache is throbbing and the child is feverish, give Belladonna 30x. Repeat the treatment frequently, as often as every fifteen minutes, until there is an improvement. If there is not a prompt response, call your homeopath or doctor.

ECZEMA

This is a condition in which the skin erupts with red spots that coalesce into smooth, orangish, flat patches. These patches often itch intensely. If it is scratched, the skin weeps and becomes rough and cracked. Eczema commonly starts in the crooks of the knees and elbows, on the cheeks, and behind the ears.

Eczema is often an allergic response, frequently to cow's milk (see pages 173-174) or to something that the skin has come in contact with. This might be the laundry detergent or fabric softener that the child's sheets or clothes have been washed in. Try using a pure soap powder and giving an extra rinse. Avoid using soap on the damaged skin. Wool often provokes eczema, so use a duvet instead of blankets and cover a sheepskin with a sheet. Buy cotton underclothes since cotton is best next to the skin.

Children with eczema are thought to be deficient in gamma-linolenic acid. They can be helped by giving evening primrose oil—start with 500 mg daily and increase until the eczema is improved (or try star flower or borage oils, which are cheaper than evening primrose).

Aromatherapy

Dry skin may be helped by applying very dilute rose, chamomile, lavender, or patchouli oil in an almond oil base.

Herbal Medicine

Eczema may be helped by putting bran or oatmeal in the baby's bath, or applying dandelion juice or breast milk to the skin. Fluid extract of goldenseal stings on contact and stains the skin yellow temporarily, but is very effective in stopping the itching and healing the condition.

In England, eczema has been successfully treated with Chinese herbal medicine.

Homeopathy

Nelson–Bach Hypercal cream may help. Eczema may require constitutional treatment from a homeopath.

FEVERS

Fevers are common in early childhood, with some children seeming to be more susceptible than others, although most get them with the infectious diseases. Sometimes children have a raised temperature for twenty-four hours for no obvious reason. It is usually highest in the evening and lowest in the morning.

A child with a temperature will have a hot head, cold hands and feet, and may be flushed. As the temperature rises, he will become either drowsy or fretful depending on the reason for the fever. A baby with a high temperature will feel hot all over. The higher the temperature, the more likely that the child will tolerate a thermometer under his arm. You should get a young baby with a temperature checked by your doctor; as he grows you will feel better able to cope with a fever by yourself.

A fever is not necessarily a bad thing; it helps to burn off the infection and shorten the illness. Acetaminophen elixir is useful to bring down a temperature that is going too high or to ease pain, but it is best, if possible, to let feverish children sleep it off. They may want to sleep all day and night, and be off their food and drink, although they should be offered drinks frequently.

Make sure that a child with a fever is lightly clad—an undershirt and diaper or underpants may be enough. If the temperature rises above 103°F (40°C), you may need to take steps to bring it down. This can be done by sponging the child with lukewarm water and allowing her to dry naturally. The cooling effect can be enhanced by adding either vinegar or lavender oil to the water. You can also try wrapping the feet in compresses soaked in cold water to which two drops of eucalyptus oil have been added. In extreme cases you may need to use a fan as well. Some children have febrile convulsions with a high temperature, alarming fits that end in sleep. These children need to be kept cool when their temperature starts to rise.

Herbal Medicine

You can bring a small child's temperature down by giving her ten drops of echinacea tincture in four ounces (120 ml) of boiled water. It may help breastfed babies if you take it yourself. Garlic perles squirted into the mouth or chewed if the child is old enough can be as effective as antibiotics. Give a minimum of six per day.

Homeopathy

A homeopathic remedy is to give ABC every fifteen minutes until there is an improvement.

On Christmas Eve, ten-year-old Alastair developed a high temperature and infected tonsils. He had lost interest in everything and sat miserably by the fire. He was encouraged to drink as many drinks containing 1-gram tablets of effervescent vitamin C as possible. He was also given lots of garlic perles throughout the day. By Christmas Day, although his tonsils were still infected, he had recovered considerably and was able to enjoy the day. He continued the treatment and was well within a couple of days.

RESUSCITATION

If a baby stops breathing, call an ambulance immediately. Give the baby gentle mouth-to-mouth resuscitation by laying her on a flat surface, tilting her head back and sealing the mouth *and* nose with your mouth. Puff air gently into the baby's lungs until the chest rises. Try to get in twenty-five breaths per minute. Continue until the baby improves or help arrives.

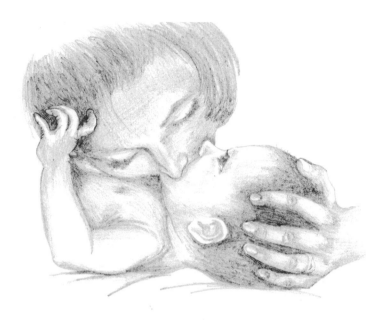

Mouth-to-mouth resuscitation on a baby. Tilt the child's head back and seal the mouth and nose with your mouth.

STICKY EYE

Babies seem prone to a condition known as sticky eye, in which the white of the eye becomes pink and pus exudes from the corners. Either one eye or both can become infected.

Breast milk squirted into the eye works wonderfully. Alternatively, you could try bathing the eye with a weak salt solution, made up of one teaspoonful of salt to one-half pint (300 ml) of cooled boiled water. Using a fresh piece each time, dip a cotton ball into the solution and wipe gently from the inner eye outward. Repeat a number of times during the day. If the condition has not cleared within three days, consult a health care practitioner.

Herbal Medicine

You could try making an infusion of eyebright or chamomile, straining it through a coffee filter, and using the liquid to bathe the eyes. Or use diluted, cold tea (add water until it is quite pale).

Homeopathy

The homeopathic remedies are Pulsatilla, Arg. nit., and Nat. phos.—try them in that order, together with the breast milk.

SUNBURN

Take great care that babies do not get sunburn, because their tender skin can burn in a very short time. Use a high factor sunscreen before taking them into the sun. If your baby's skin is burned, use Nelson–Bach AfterSun cream or another ointment for burns.

SURGERY (BABIES)

It can be a horrible experience to have your child operated on. It is always worth asking an alternative practitioner whether there is any way of remedying the complaint without surgery; for example, a child with frequent ear infection may not need to have tubes inserted into the eardrum if treated with cranial osteopathy to improve drainage of fluid from the inner ear.

Homeopathy

If surgery is unavoidable, the following homeopathic remedies are advocated by Jane Arnold of the Active Birth Movement in her booklet *Homeopathy for Pregnancy, Childbirth and Infancy*. If there is a tendency to bleed, give Phosphorus before surgery. For cut nerve endings, give Hypericum. For fear (yours or the childs), give Aconite, one dose before and one after surgery, followed by Arnica and Hypericum alternately, two doses of each, every day for several days. You may want to consult a homeopath about an antidote to a general anesthetic.

TANTRUMS AND IRRITABILITY

Children in a really bad mood can be cheered up by being placed in a bath with a drop or two of clary sage oil in it. They may also be soothed and calmed by a gentle back massage. Massaging your child can help relieve the feeling of frustration you may feel at dealing with a child that seems determined to be unreasonable.

TEETHING

Teething is notorious for upsetting babies. There is a wide variation in the age at which the first tooth appears, and it may cause trouble long before it finally shows as a thin line in the gum. The tooth appears as a bulge under the skin and often seems to rise and recede as the gums swell in response to the small sharp edge being forced through them. It is this stage that seems to cause the most pain. Each child varies, but the teething process can be accompanied by lots of crying and fretfulness, red cheeks, night waking, and drooling. In some cases it results in diarrhea and diaper rash and even apparent coughs and colds. It should not raise the temperature, but if your baby has a fever too, take the child to your doctor.

Water-filled teethers or rubber teething rings will help those babies who become frantic to bite on things. Others, however, cannot bear anything to touch the gums and may need acetaminophen elixir to help with the pain. Nelson–Bach makes a special preparation of chamomilla granules for teething suitable for a baby who is angry and crying, screams if put down, and has green diarrhea. Also try Rescue Remedy, for both yourself and the baby. Rubbing the gums with ice, brandy, or lemon juice may help ease the pain.

Aromatherapy

A teething baby may be soothed by a drop of lavender or chamomile oil put onto the sheet near its head.

Homeopathy

Try ABC to start, if necessary followed by one of the following remedies. For teething that results in a fever with one cheek that is especially pale or bright red, give Aconite. For a baby that is flushed, especially if there is a tendency to convulsions, give Belladonna. For teething that makes the baby weepy, whiny, and changeable, give Pulsatilla.

THRUSH

Babies sometimes get thrush inside their mouths. It shows as stubborn white patches on the cheeks. They can be removed by squirting the liquid from garlic perles onto the affected parts. A homeopathic remedy is to give Borax or Candida.

Thrush also appears on the baby's bottom as a distinctive form of diaper rash that develops in islands. This can be treated topically (see pages 186–187) and also systemically, by giving the child two garlic perles three times a day, until it clears. Recurrent thrush may mean that you should consider treatment from a homeopath.

VOMITING

Babies are often a little bit sick—and a little goes a long way. Some babies seem to enjoy feeding and then sending the surplus back, while seeming quite happy and gaining weight. Some are decidedly more prone to spitting up in this way than others. It creates a lot of mess and washing, but there is nothing wrong with the baby. You can prevent your child from this tendency by having acupuncture treatments during the fourteenth and twenty-sixth weeks of pregnancy. Be aware of the possibility that food intolerance may be causing vomiting when you start weaning.

There are two kinds of vomiting that should be taken seriously. The first is due to infection, when a baby suddenly and repeatedly vomits large amounts. She may be unable to keep anything down and may have diarrhea as well. Give Pedialyte to drink (see page 185) and seek help if the baby vomits more than two complete feeds consecutively. Meadowsweet infusion can help to settle the stomach.

The other type of serious vomiting is due to pyloric stenosis. This either starts suddenly or builds up gradually and consists of the baby vomiting following feeds so forcefully that vomit shoots out of the mouth and lands some feet away; it is known as projectile vomiting. It is most common in boys and generally starts after three weeks. Treatment is essential either with surgery or from a cranial osteopath.

Endnotes

Chapter 3: Planning for Pregnancy

1. I. P. Gillies and M. Wakefield, "Smoking in Pregnancy," *Current Obstetrics and Gynaecology* 3, No. 3 (September 1993): 157–61.
2. S. K. Rosevear, D. W. Holt, T. D. Lee, et al., "Smoking and Decreased Fertilization Rates in Vitro," *Lancet* 340, No. 8829 (14 November 1992): 1195–96.
3. N. Wald, J. Sneddon, J. Densom, C. Frost, and R. Stone, "Prevention of Neural Tube Defects: Results of the Medical Research Council Vitamin Study," *Lancet* 338 (1991): 131–37.

Chapter 6: Preparing Yourself for Pregnancy and Birth

1. A. E. Czeizel, "Prevention of Congenital Abnormalities by Periconceptual Multi-vitamin supplements," *British Medical Journal* 306, No. 6893 (19 June 1993): 1645–48.
2. *Nutrition Review* 50, No. 8 (1992): 233–36.
3. American College of Obstetrics and Gynecology Committee on Obstetrics, "Vitamin A Supplementation during Pregnancy," *International Journal of Gynecology and Obstetrics* 40 (1993): 175.

Chapter 7: An A–Z of Possible Problems and Their Remedies

1. Althea Seaver, "Feeling Fine: Avoiding Some Common Discomforts in Preganancy," *Midwifery Today*, No. 21 (Spring 1992): 22–24.
2. D. Alyosio and P. Penacchioni, *Obstetrics and Gynaecology* 80, No. 5 (November 1992): 852–54.
3. V. Sahakian, D. Rouse, S. Sipes, *Obstetrics and Gyanecology* 78, No. 1 (July 1991): 33–36.
4. A. Neri, G. Sabah, and Z. Samra, *Acta Obstetrica et Gynecologica* 72, No. 1 (January 1993): 17–19.

Chapter 9: When Labor Is Not Straightforward

1. The due date is usually held to be forty weeks from conception, although in fact, left to itself, the true average length of pregnancy is forty-one weeks and one day. This explains why roughly 30 percent of babies arrive before the due date and 70 percent afterward.
2. Two recent studies suggest that this can be an effective and safe method of inducing labor that works for two-thirds of women within three days of the procedure. H. A. Allot and C. R. Palmer "Sweeping the Membranes: A Valid Procedure in Stimulating the Onset of Labour?" *British Journal of Obstetrics and Gynaecology* 100, No. 10 (October 1993): 893–900; J. M. Grant, "Sweeping of the Membranes in Prolonged Pregnancy," *British Journal of Obstetrics and Gynaecology* 100, No. 10 (October 1993): 18–24.
3. E. Burns and K. Greenish, "Pooling Information," *Nursing Times* 89, No. 8 (February 1993): 47–49.

Chapter 11: Breastfeeding

1. J. M. Alexander, A. M. Grant, and M. J. Campbell, *British Medical Journal* 304, No. 6833 (18 April 1992): 1030–32.
2. G. Dewan, C. Glazner, and M. Tunstall, "Postnatal Pain: A Neglected Area," *British Journal of Midwifery* 1, No. 2 (June 1993): 63–66.
3. W. L. Nicholson, "The Use of Nipple Shields by Breast-feeding Women," *Australian College of Midwives Incorporated Journal* 6, No. 2 (June 1993): 18–24.

4. J. Lloyd, *Australian Lactation Consultants Association News* 3, No. 2 (August 1992): 3–4.

Chapter 12: You and Your Baby

1. E. Adamson-Macedo, "Massage and Midwifery," *Midwifery Matters* 56 (Spring 1993): 5–6.
2. L. Paterson, "Baby Massage in the Neonatal Unit," *Paediatric Nursing* 4, No. 23 (1990): 19–21; and J. Russell, "Touch and Infant Massage,"*Paediatric Nursing* 5, No. 3 (April 1993): 8–11.

Suggested Reading

GENERAL

Arms, Suzanne. *Immaculate Deception II: Birth and Beyond.* Berkeley, Calif.: Celestial Arts, 1993.

Balaskas, Janet, and Arthur Balaskas. *New Life.* London, Sidgwick & Jackson, 1983

Balaskas, Janet, and Yehudi Gordon. *The Encyclopedia of Pregnancy and Birth.* London: Macdonald, 1989.

Bastien, Alison Parra. "Postpartum Rituals: Honoring the Mother," *Midwifery Today* 20, No. 22 (Summer 1992): 32–33.

Boston Women's Health Book Collective. *Our Bodies, Ourselves: Updated and Expanded for the '90s.* New York: Simon & Schuster, 1992.

Castro, Miranda. *Homeopathy for Mother and Baby: A Guide to Pregnancy, Birth and the Post-natal Years.* London: Macmillan, 1992.

Davies, Stephen, and Alan Stewart. *Nutritional Medicine: The Drug-Free Guide to Better Family Health.* New York: Avon, 1990.

Harper, Barbara. *Gentle Birth Choices: A Guide to Making Informed Decisions.* Rochester, Vt.: Healing Arts Press, 1994.

Hawkridge, Caroline. *Living with Endometriosis.* London: Vermilion, 1996.

Hewitt, James. *The Complete Relaxation Book.* London: Rider, 1982.

Kitzinger, Sheila. *Women as Mothers.* New York: Random House, 1980.

———. *Your Baby, Your Way: Making Pregnancy Decisions and Birth Plans.* New York: Pantheon Books, 1987.

———. *Homebirth: The Essential Guide to Giving Birth Outside of the Hospital.* London: Dorling Kindersley, 1991.

———. *The Complete Book of Pregnancy and Childbirth,* rev. ed. New York: Alfred A. Knopf, 1996.

Lawless, Julia. *The Encyclopedia of Essential Oils.* Shaftesbury, Dorset: Element, 1992.

Leboyer, Frederick. *Birth without Violence.* New York: Alfred A. Knopf, 1975. Reprint, Rochester, Vt.: Healing Arts Press, 1995.

McIntyre, Anne. *The Complete Woman's Herbal.* London: Gaia, 1996.

———. *The Complete Floral Healer.* London: Gaia, 1996.

Reynolds, Jan. *Mother and Child: Visions of Parenting from Indigenous Cultures.* Rochester, Vt.: Inner Traditions, 1997.

Tang, Stephen. *Chinese Herbal Medicine.* London: Rich and Craze Piatkus, 1995.

Tiran, Denise. *Complementary Therapies for Pregnancy and Birth.* London: Bailliere Tindall, 1994.

Wagner, Marsden. *The Birth Machine.* Philadelphia: Temple Univ. Press, 1993.

Welford, Heather. *A–Z of Feeding in the First Year.* London: Unwin, 1988.

Wesson, Nicky. *Home Birth.* London: Vermilion, 1996.

Westcott, Patsy. *Alternative Health Care for Women: A Woman's Guide to Self-help Treatments and Natural Therapies.* Rochester, Vt.: Healing Arts Press, 1988.

ACUPUNCTURE AND ACUPRESSURE

Kenyon, Julian. *Acupressure Techniques: A Self-Help Guide,* rev. ed. Rochester, Vt.: Healing Arts Press, 1988.

Chaitow, Leon, N.D., D.O. *The Acupuncture Treatment of Pain.* Rochester, Vt.: Healing Arts Press, 1990.

AROMATHERAPY AND BACH FLOWER REMEDIES

England, Allison. *Aromatherapy for Mother and Baby: Natural Healing with Essential Oils During Pregnancy and Early Motherhood.* Rochester, Vt.: Healing Arts Press, 1994.

Mazzarella, Barbara. *Bach Flower Remedies for Children.* Rochester, Vt.: Healing Arts Press, 1997.

Scheffer, Mechthild. *Bach Flower Therapy: Theory and Practice.* Rochester, Vt.: Healing Arts Press, 1992.

Tisserand, Maggie. *Aromatherapy for Women,* rev. ed. Rochester, Vt.: Healing Arts Press, 1996.

Wildwood, Chrissie. *The Encyclopedia of Aromatherapy.* Rochester, Vt.: Healing Arts Press, 1997.

HERBAL MEDICINE

Gladstar, Rosemary. *Herbal Healing for Women: Simple Home Remedies for Women of All Ages.* New York: Simon & Schuster, 1993.

Hoffmann, David. *The New Holistic Herbal.* Rockport, Mass.: Element Books, 1991.

Levy, Juliette de Bairacli. *The Illustrated Herbal Handbook.* London: Faber, 1982.

McIntyre, Michael. *Herbal Medicine for Everyone.* London: Penguin, 1990.

Theiss, Barbara, and Peter Theiss. *The Family Herbal: A Guide to Natural Health Care for Yourself and Your Children from Europe's Leading Herbalists*. Rochester, Vt.: 1993.

Tyler, Varro, E., Ph.D. *The Honest Herbal: A Sensible Guide to the Use of Herbs and Related Remedies*, 3rd ed. New York: Pharmaceutical Products Press, 1993.

Weed, Susun. *The Wise Woman Herbal for the Childbearing Year*. Woodstock, N.Y.: Ash Tree Publishing, 1992.

HOMEOPATHY

Arnold, Jane. *Homeopathy for Pregnancy, Childbirth, and Infancy*. Manuscript.

Gibson, Sheila, M.D., and Robin Gibson, M.D. *Homeopathy for Everyone*. London: Penguin, 1991.

Hayfield, Robin. *The Family Homeopath: Safe, Natural, and Effective Health Care for You and Your Children*. Rochester, Vt.: Healing Arts Press, 1994.

Morgan, Lyle W., Ph.D. *Homeopathy and Your Child: A Parent's Guide to Homeopathic Treatment from Infancy through Adolescence*. Rochester, Vt.: Healing Arts Press, 1992.

MASSAGE

Hudson, Clare Maxwell. *The Complete Book of Massage*. London: Dorling Kindersley, 1988.

Russel, Stephen, and Yehudi Gordon. *Massage for Life*. Manuscript.

Johari, Harish. *Ayurvedic Massage: Traditional Indian Techniques for Balancing Body and Mind*. Rochester, Vt.: Healing Arts Press, 1997.

REFLEXOLOGY

Dougans, Inge, and Suzanne Ellis. *Art of Reflexology*. Rockport, Mass.: Element Books, 1992.

Kunz, Kevin, and Barbara Kunz. *Complete Guide to Foot Reflexology*. London: Thorsons, 1984.

Wills, Pauline. *The Reflexology Manual: An Easy-to-Use Illustrated Guide to the Healing Zones of the Hands and Feet*. Rochester, Vt.: Healing Arts Press, 1995.

Resources

Academy of Certified Birth Educators (ACBE) and Labor Support
Professionals
2001 E. Prairie Circle, Suite 1, Olathe, KS 66062
(913) 782-5116; (800) 444-8223
Offers courses on childbirth education and Doula Training.

The Bradley Method
P. O. Box 5224, Sherman Oaks, CA 91413-5224
(800) 4-A-BIRTH
www.Bradleybirth.com
Provides free national directory of Bradley Method of Childbirth Educators and informational package. Sponsors workshops and certifies childbirth educators.

American College of Nurse-Midwives (ACNM)
818 Connecticut Avenue NW, Suite 900, Washington, DC 20006
(202) 728-9860

into@acnm.org
Founded in 1955 to establish and maintain standards for the practice of nurse-midwifery. National headquarters provides information about nurse-midwifery and referrals to nurse-midwives. For referrals in your area, call toll-free, twenty-four hours a day: 888-MIDWIFE.

American Society of Psychoprophylaxis in Obstetrics (ASPO Lamaze)
1840 Wilson Boulevard, Suite 204, Arlington, VA 22201
(800) 368-4404
Introduced the Lamaze method to the United States and continues to offer classes and certification for childbirth educators.

Cascade Healthcare & Birth and Life Bookstore
141 Commercial Street N.E., Salem, OR 97301
(800) 443-9942
Sells home birth supplies and educational books and materials available by mail order. Now incorporates the Birth and Life Bookstore, which has the largest available selection of books and videos about pregnancy, birth, parenting, and midwifery.

Cesarean/Support, Education, and Concern (C/SEC)
22 Forest Road, Framingham, MA 01701
(508) 877-8266
Offers information and support for cesarean prevention and vaginal birth after cesarean (VBAC) as well as nationwide training workshops for childbirth educators. Representatives available for telephone consultations in your area.

Co-Creations for Joyful Births, Inc.
290 North Main Street, Suite 8, Ashland, OR 97520
(541) 488-3446
Offers Doula services, childbirth education classes, and early parenting classes.

Informed Homebirth/Informed Birth and Parenting
P. O. Box 3675, Ann Arbor, MI 48106
(313) 662-6857
Provides information on alternatives in birth, parenting, and education. Referrals to midwives, childbirth educators, and labor assistants. National conference on Waldorf (Steiner) education and home schooling.

International Association of Parents and Professionals for Safe Alternatives in Childbirth (NAPSAC)
Route 1, Box 646, Marble Hill, MO 63764
(573) 238-2010
NAPSAC publishes books and pamphlets supporting the alternative birth movement and offers an international directory of alternative birth services.

International Childbirth Education Association (ICEA)
P. O. Box 20048, Mineapolis MN 55420-0048
(612) 854-8660
Certifies childbirth educators and publishes a journal and a catalog of books, pamphlets, and videos on childbirth and family-centered maternity care.

International Lactation Consultant Association (ILCA)
200 North Michigan Avenue, Suite 300, Chicago, IL 60601
(312) 541-1710
Provides support and up-to-date information about breastfeeding.

La Leche League International (LLLI)
1400 N. Meacham Road, P. O. Box 4079, Schaumburg, IL 60168-4079
(847) 519-7730; Hotline: 800-LA LECHE
Call the hotline between 9 A.M. and 3 P.M. (CST) for breastfeeding help or a referral to a local LLLI support group. LLLI also publishes many informative books on breastfeeding.

Midwifery Today Magazine

P. O. Box 2672, Eugene, OR 97402

(800) 743-0974

Geared toward birth professionals but has excellent articles about home birth, natural childbirth, and midwifery that parents will also find useful.

National Women's Health Network

514 Tenth Street NW, Suite 400, Washington, DC 20004

(202) 347-1140

Monitors federal policies that affect women's health, especially in the area of reproductive rights and environmental and occupational health. A newsletter and other publications are available.

ACUPUNCTURE

American Academy of Medical Acupuncture (AAMA)

Administrative Offices

5820 Wilshire Boulevard #500, Los Angeles, CA 90036

(800) 521-2262

The sole physician-only professional acupuncture society in North America. Provides information to the public and referrals to practitioners who are members. Information is available on-line at http://www.medicalacupuncture.org/index.htm. This site also provides links to other sites of interest.

National Acupuncture and Oriental Medicine Alliance

14637 Starr Road SE, Olalla, WA 98359

(206) 851-6896

Membership organization that provides referrals and literature.

AROMATHERAPY

American AromaTherapy Association (AATA)
P. O. Box 3243, South Pasadena, CA 91031
Holds an annual convention and offers educational guidelines and networking for practitioners.

The American Society for Phytotherapy and Aromatherapy International, Inc.
P. O. Box 3679, South Pasadena, CA 91031

AromaVéra, Inc.
P. O. Box 3609, Culver City, CA 90231
(800) 669-9514; (310) 280-0407
Imports more than seventy essential oils. Purchases directly from producers. Carries aromatic diffusers and an extensive line of aromatherapy products available by mail order.

BACH FLOWER REMEDIES

Ellon USA
644 Merrick Road, Lynbrook, NY 11563
(800) 4BE-CALM; (516) 593-2206
Offers original Bach Flower Remedies by mail order.

HERBAL MEDICINE

Herb Research Foundation
1007 Pearl Street, Suite 200, Boulder, CO 80302
(303) 449-2265; Fax: (303) 449-7849
An independent nonprofit organization dedicated to providing reliable scientific botanical data for its members, the public, and the media.

HOMEOPATHY

Boiron/USA
6 Campus Boulevard, Building A, Newton Square, PA 19073
(610) 325-7464; (800) BLUE-TUBE

Nelson–Bach USA
Wilmington Technology Park
100 Research Drive, Wilmington, MA 01887-4406
Manufacture and sell homeopathic remedies.

Homeopathic Educational Services
2124 Kittredge Street, Berkeley, CA 94704
(510) 649-0294; (800) 359-9051 (orders only)
mail@homeopathic.com
Extensive list of books on homeopathy and related health issues; remedy kits. Free catalog.

International Foundation for Homeopathy (IFH)
P. O. Box 7, Edmonds, WA 98020
(206) 776-4147; Fax: (206) 776-1499
A nonprofit organization dedicated to the education of professional homeopaths according to the highest standards of classical homeopathy. Activities include professional courses, an annual conference, and a bimonthly magazine. Referrals to graduates of the IFH professional course will be provided with a SASE.

National Center for Homeopathy (NCH)
801 North Fairfax Street, Suite 306, Alexandria, VA 22314
(703) 548-7790; Fax: (703) 548-7792
nchinfo@igc.apc.org
A nonprofit organization promoting homeopathy in the United States through education, publication, research, and membership services.

Membership is $40/year and includes the monthly magazine *Homeopathy Today* and the annual directory of practitioners, study groups, and resources. An information packet, which includes the directory, is available to nonmembers for $6. The directory is also available at http://www.homeopathic.org.

Standard Homeopathic Company
210 West 131 Street
Box 61067, Los Angeles, CA 90061
(800) 624-9659; (213) 321-4284
Manufactures a full line of homeopathic medicines in various dosage forms, including tincture, dilution, pellets, and tablets.

HYPNOTHERAPY

American Council of Hypnotism Examiners
700 South Central Avenue, Glendale, CA 91204
(818) 242-1159
Provides information about hypnotherapy.

OSTEOPATHY

United States Directory of Osteopathic Physicians
On-line directory of more than 20,000 osteopathic physicians: http://www.rscom/osteous.

Index